# An Eye for the Sky

# PRAISE FOR THE BOOK

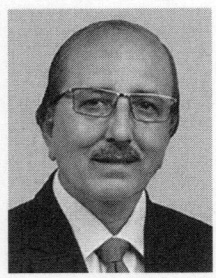

**Padma Shri Professor Jagat Ram**
Past director, Post Graduate Institute of Medical Education and Research (PGIMER), Chandigarh.

Dr Suresh K. Pandey was my student at PGIMER, Chandigarh in 1995–97. *An Eye for the Sky* motivates everyone to aim high and work hard to utilize their full potential. This is an excellent resource for each and every lay reader as well as medical professional. Dr Pandey has shared his passionate journey which began with living in poverty in a village, studying in the light of a lantern, and harbouring an intense desire to become an eye doctor. He has shared his trials and tribulations while studying medicine in India and while training abroad in the USA and Australia. He also shared various challenges that came along his way as well as the golden formulae for success. His memoir gives a clear message: if he can do it, you can too.

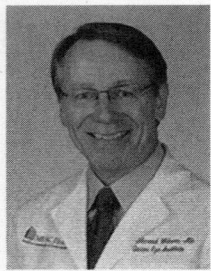

**Professor M. Edward Wilson**
Storm Eye Institute, Medical University of South Carolina, Charleston, USA

*An Eye for the Sky* inspires each and every reader to keep working till their goal is achieved. He was one of the dedicated fellows of the Late Professor David J. Apple (Apple Korps) and also worked under my guidance from 1998 to 2001 at the Storm Eye Institute. He completed the important work of writing and editing *Pediatric Cataract Surgery* which was published by the world-famous publisher Lippincott, Williams and Wilkins. Dr Pandey and his wife Dr Vidushi Sharma are living the life values that every reader, medical student, and trainee medical student can learn from.

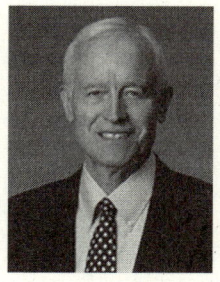

**Professor Randall J. Olson**
Chairman, John A. Moran Eye Center, University of Utah, Salt Lake City, USA

*An Eye for the Sky* written by my fellow Dr Suresh K. Pandey guides each reader to reach their destination while overcoming the obstacles in the way. In the chapters of this book, Dr Pandey has shared his life journey and his struggles from childhood to become a high-volume ophthalmic surgeon. He has shared the story of his grandfather, who was considered a messiah of sight and was a huge inspiration for him to become an eye surgeon. He has also shared several interesting anecdotes from his time of pursuing ophthalmology training in India, America and Australia. This memoir would be an interesting read for every reader, particularly medical students, young doctors and medical professionals, and would motivate them to become caring and compassionate doctors.

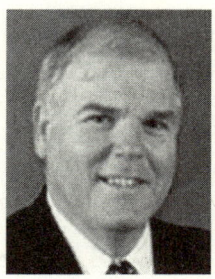

**Dr E. John Milverton**
Chairman, Intraocular Implant Unit, Sydney Eye Hospital, University of Sydney, Australia

*An Eye for the Sky* is a very inspiring memoir, where Dr Pandey has shared his mantras for success while facing life's many curveballs. Dr Suresh K. Pandey and Dr Vidushi Sharma worked under my guidance at Sydney Eye Hospital, Australia, during the years 2003 and 2004. They learned the art of ocular microsurgery and also published several articles on eye surgery, eye research journals and presented research papers at eye conferences. Dr Pandey's memoir is a milestone for every reader looking for motivation and will prove to be very useful for coaching students, medical students and young doctors.

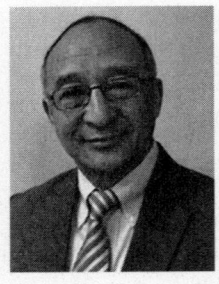

I congratulate Dr Suresh K. Pandey for the publication of his excellent memoir *An Eye for the Sky*. I had the opportunity to meet and interact with him several times during international ophthalmology conferences. His spouse Dr Vidushi Sharma was my student at Dr R.P. Centre for Ophthalmic Sciences, AIIMS, New Delhi. This book is a most inspirational account for overcoming life's obstacles and will help guide medical students in becoming successful doctors and will also play an important role in strengthening the doctor–patient relationship.

**Padma Shri Professor Jeewan Singh Titiyal**
Director, Dr Rajendra Prasad Institute of Ophthalmology, All India Institute of Ophthalmology (AIIMS), New Delhi

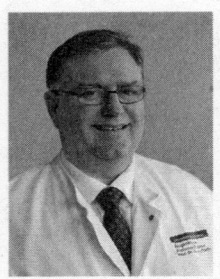

*An Eye on the Sky* is an excellent memoir written by Dr Suresh K. Pandey, one of the 'Apple Korps'. It is sure to inspire all its readers to excel in life and realize their complete potential against all odds.

**Professor Gerd U. Auffarth**
Head of the David J. Apple Center for Vision Research Chairman, University of Heidelberg, Germany

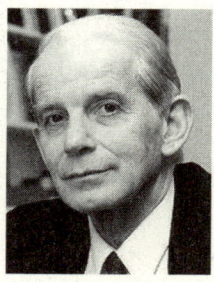

I would like to congratulate my fellow Dr Suresh K. Pandey and Dr Vidushi Sharma for publishing Dr Pandey's inspiring memoir—a must-read for every medical professional!

**Professor Frank A. Billson**
University of Sydney, Australia

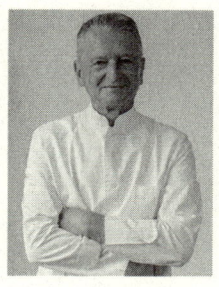

*An Eye for the Sky* provides insight into the inspiring journey of Dr Suresh K. Pandey from a dusty village to becoming a docpreneur. This memoir is a timely contribution to inspire all readers, especially medical professionals. I congratulate Dr Pandey on this excellent memoir that will be helpful for young doctors to start their own medical practices and earn patients' trust.

**Dr Lucio Buratto**
Centro Ambrosiano Oftalmico
(CAMO), Milan, Italy

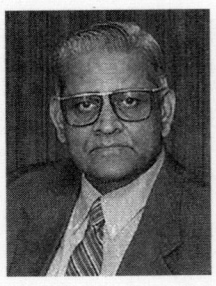

*An Eye for the Sky* is an excellent memoir written by Dr Suresh K. Pandey to motivate his readers—medical students, doctors-in-training and young doctors—to do well professionally. The author has shared the many trials and tribulations he faced on his journey from a small village to the magnificent world stage of ophthalmology. This book will be very inspirational for every reader, particularly young doctors.

**Padma Shri**
**Dr S. S. Badrinath**
Sankara Nethralaya,
Chennai

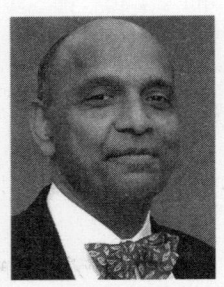

*An Eye for the Sky* is an excellent read, sure to prove immensely helpful for every medical professional. I congratulate Dr. Suresh K. Pandey for publishing this excellent memoir and for sharing valuable lessons for young doctors.

**Padma Shri Dr Gullapalli**
**Nageswara Rao**
Director Emeritus,
L.V. Prasad Eye Institute,
Hyderabad

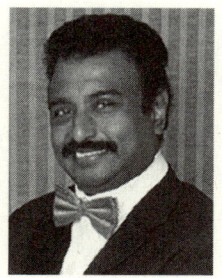

*An Eye for the Sky* is a must-read memoir for every medical professional. I congratulate Dr Suresh K. Pandey for bringing out his excellent book and sharing every step of his journey from becoming a doctor to a doctorpreneur. An excellent book for all readers, especially doctors and medical professionals.

**Padma Shri Dr Natarajan Sundaram**
Chairman, Aditya Jyot
Eye Hospital, Chennai

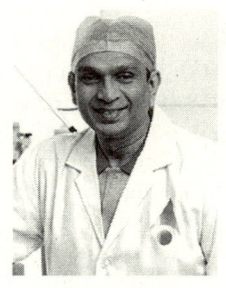

*An Eye for the Sky* is one of the best reads for young doctors. It reveals a toolkit to becoming a successful medical entrepreneur. I am sure the book will be immensely useful for young medical professionals. Dr Suresh K. Pandey deserves many congratulations for the publication of his moving memoir.

**Dr Amar Agarwal**
Director, Dr Agarwal
Group of Eye Hospital,
Chennai, India

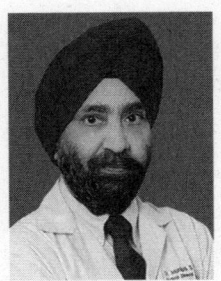

*An Eye for the Sky* is an excellent read for every medical student, doctor and health professional. My hearty congratulations to Dr Suresh K. Pandey!

**Padma Shri Dr Mahipal S. Sachdev**
Centre for Sight Group of Eye Hospitals, New Delhi, India

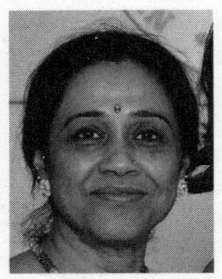

My congratulations to Dr Suresh K. Pandey, an alumnus of Netaji Subhash Chandra Bose Medical College, Jabalpur, for publishing his outstanding memoir, *An Eye for the Sky*. He is one of the few practising eye doctors in India to have contributed to research, education and health awareness in such a large measure. Through his own remarkable story, the book documents the fundamentals of what makes a person achieve meaningful success in any field of their choosing. I am sure this book will inspire every reader, especially NEET coaching students, medical students, young doctors and medical professionals.

**Dr Geeta Guin**
Dean, Netaji Subhash Chandra Bose Medical College, Jabalpur, Madhya Pradesh

# An Eye for the Sky

## How an Eye Surgeon Helped Millions Dare to Dream

## Dr Suresh K. Pandey

MBBS, MS (Ophthalmology, PGIMER, Chandigarh)
Ant. Segment Fellowship (USA and Australia)
Director, SuVi Eye Hospital and Lasik Laser Centre,
Kota, Rajasthan, India
Visiting Assistant Professor, John A. Moran Eye Center,
University of Utah, Salt Lake City, Utah, USA

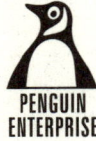

PENGUIN
ENTERPRISE

An imprint of Penguin Random House

PENGUIN ENTERPRISE

Penguin Enterprise is an imprint of the Penguin Random House group of companies
whose addresses can be found at global.penguinrandomhouse.com

Published by Penguin Random House India Pvt. Ltd
4th Floor, Capital Tower 1, MG Road,
Gurugram 122 002, Haryana, India

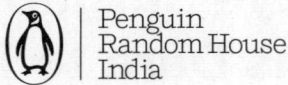

Penguin
Random House
India

First published in Penguin Enterprise by Penguin Random House India 2024

Copyright © Dr Suresh K. Pandey 2024

All rights reserved

10 9 8 7 6 5 4 3 2 1

ISBN 9780143459033

Typeset in Baskerville
Printed at Thomson Press India Ltd, New Delhi

www.penguin.co.in

MIX
Paper | Supporting
responsible forestry
FSC® C010615

*My grandparents, Late Dr Kamta Prasad Pandey and*
*Late Smt Ram Shringari Devi, and parents,*
*Late Shri Kameshwar Prasad Pandey and Smt Maya Pandey,*
*who taught me by example how to lead a meaningful life.*
*Dr Vidushi Sharma, my wife, who has walked alongside me.*
*Ishita, my daughter, for her love and for understanding*
*Papa's passion for writing.*
*Thousands of patients in India and overseas*
*who placed their trust in my hands.*

*And a destiny that took me to unimaginable peaks . . .*

## An Ophthalmologist's Prayer

Give me work when I am young
Let there be no unexpected complications on the operation table
Let no unexpected guest (vitreous) appear during my cataract surgery
Let me not cross a point of no return during an operation
Let my skilful hands not make me arrogant
Keep me away from the temptations of wealth
Let the invisible enemies, the microbes, not infect the patient's eye
Give me the wisdom to quit in time
Give me good health to enjoy the evening of my life.

# Contents

# Foreword

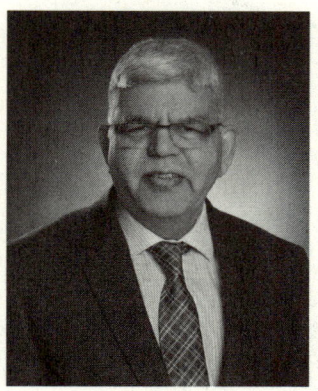

Doctors are the backbone of our society, serving as guardians of health and well-being. They possess the remarkable ability to alleviate suffering, cure illnesses and rescue lives from the brink of despair. The transformative impact they have on individuals is immeasurable, and their unwavering compassion and empathy are what endear them to the public. Through active listening, deep understanding and the delivery of precise treatments, doctors build the foundation of trust and confidence upon which their patients rely.

Yet, success in any field is not a mere download away, like a convenient app on a smartphone, that instantly alters the course of one's life. It is a demanding and often treacherous journey, riddled with countless obstacles, difficulties and unexpected detours. When confronted with these challenges, most people choose to retreat or, worse, give up entirely. However, a select few rise to the occasion, determined to surmount any difficulty in their path. Dr Suresh K. Pandey, my dedicated student, stands out as a shining example of the latter. His journey was anything but smooth, marred by numerous hurdles, yet none could overshadow the brilliance of his dream. Driven by unwavering conviction, he has exemplified that those with a clear vision for their goals and an unrelenting passion to turn that vision into reality, can overcome any obstacle and achieve even the loftiest of goals.

Dr Pandey's life has been a testament to going the extra mile, facing challenges head-on and pushing one's limits. His resilience and determination can be succinctly described as 'unstoppable'. A devoted student of ophthalmology, he constantly strives to learn and reinvent himself, keeping the flame of curiosity and knowledge alive.

His memoir, titled *An Eye for the Sky*, embodies the multifaceted persona of Dr Pandey. Within its pages, one discovers not only the accomplished doctor but also the prolific researcher, dedicated teacher, inspirational motivator and innovative entrepreneur. This book serves as a wellspring of inspiration, drawing from his life experiences. It demonstrates how spirituality, faith, intuition and empathy can seamlessly intertwine with the worlds of medicine and science, creating a harmonious symphony of healing and discovery.

Dr Pandey's intention is clear: to inspire and motivate readers of all backgrounds, from aspiring medical students to young doctors and healthcare professionals, through his memoir. His roots trace back to a small village, where basic amenities were scarce and education was a distant dream. Dr Pandey's early education was marked by arduous journeys, walking several kilometres to school and studying by the dim light of an oil lantern due to the lack of electricity. His perseverance saw him through medical school, often surviving on just one meal a day and saving every penny he could scrounge. His life journey is a testament to dedication and determination in the pursuit of a dream—a dream that would see him become a distinguished doctor.

The pages of his memoir unfold an awe-inspiring success story, one that entails overcoming every obstacle life tosses in one's path. Dr Pandey's motivation transcends the personal realm; he is driven to help the underprivileged by restoring the gift of sight to countless patients. His care, compassion and unwavering commitment to humanity shine through in his efforts to make a difference in the world.

Dr Pandey's remarkable journey spans across three different countries—India, the USA and Australia. He shares the invaluable lessons, tips and tricks that empowered him to establish SuVi Eye Hospital in Kota alongside his wife, Dr Vidushi Sharma, despite having no prior entrepreneurial experience. The book is brimming with captivating stories, insightful anecdotes and life lessons, creating a captivating narrative that imparts wisdom on how to live a truly fulfilling life.

I have no doubt that this book will serve as a well of inspiration for every reader, whether they are NEET coaching students, medical aspirants, young doctors, seasoned medical professionals, or anyone else in search of an inspirational narrative, from any corner of the globe. Dr Suresh Pandey and his family have my heartfelt best wishes as they continue to make a positive impact on the world.

**Professor (Dr) Amod Gupta,**
**(Awarded Padma Shri by the President of India)**
Professor Emeritus Ophthalmology, Former Dean, Former Chief, Advanced Eye Centre, Post Graduate Institute of Medical Education and Research (PGIMER), Chandigarh, India.

# Prologue

## My Journey from Mohna to the
## Magnificent Stage of Ophthalmology

My prayer has been answered
I am blessed to be in my profession,
I am fifty-five years old; helping restore the gift of sight, my passion,
And full of happy memories,
My life overflows with hidden treasures which no authority can tax;
No one can ever know that I envy my destiny.

I was born in a small village Mohna, situated near Rawatbhata, district Chittorgarh, Rajasthan. I studied under the light of a lantern and walked five kilometers barefoot to attend my school. I had an intense desire to become an eye doctor. I faced countless obstacles and challenges in my journey and even felt very depressed at times. However, I overcame these difficulties with passion, planning, perseverance, practice and a positive attitude. After completing my medical training at NSCB Medical College Jabalpur and ophthalmology training at Post Graduate Institute of Medical Education and Research (PGIMER), Chandigarh,

I moved to the USA in June 1998. I totally immersed myself in ophthalmology research at Storm Eye Institute. From Mohna to the magnificent stage of ophthalmology, my journey through the uncharted territory of a medical career was filled with trials and tribulations.

The year 2002, after four years of hard work, I was greeted with great recognition for my research work on the global stage of ophthalmology. I spent several months performing research and preparing articles and a video on Intraocular Lens Opacification. This work was done at the Centre for Research on Ocular Therapeutics and Biodevices, Storm Eye Institute, Charleston, USA, in collaboration with eye surgeons from Europe, the USA and Australia. My research answered the causes of the cloudiness (opacification) of the intraocular lens (IOL) several years after successful cataract surgery. Ophthalmic surgeons were getting hundreds of patients with complaints of hazy vision after successful cataract surgery and lens implantation. They were unable to detect the cause of the cloudiness of these intraocular lenses. Some of these eye surgeons got confused with the hazy posterior capsule and also performed the Nd: Yag Laser posterior capsulotomy which did not result in improving the vision in any way. Some of them were sued by patients for their inability to explain the cause of the cloudiness of the implant which had helped them regain their vision. A few surgeons explanted these opacified IOLs and sent them to Professor David J. Apple for detailed evaluation and research. I, together with Dr Liliana Werner, examined these explanted intraocular lenses and found that they had calcium deposition on the surface. We recorded a video where I explained the procedure and presented my seminal research, which won me the prestigious American Society of Cataract and Refractive Surgery (ASCRS) Film Festival Award (2002), the European Society of Cataract and Refractive Surgeons (ESCRS) Film Festival Award (2002) and Best of the Show Video Award during the American Academy of Ophthalmology (AAO)

Conference in 2002. I received a letter of congratulations from AAO and was invited to attend the award ceremony for the Best of Show Video Award.

I reached Orlando, USA, in October 2002 at the annual meeting of the American Academy of Ophthalmology (AAO). There were dignitaries from all around the world: 18,000 ophthalmologists, vision scientists, residents, and students from across the globe in the same room. The meeting was one of the largest of its kind in the world, featuring significant advances in the field of ophthalmology, and bringing together clinicians, vision scientists and researchers from over 110 countries. I had already attended the meeting a few times before this occasion.

But today was no ordinary day. There was an award up for grabs: A Best-of-the-Show Video Award by the American Academy of Ophthalmology. Two weeks ago, I received a letter saying that my video on intraocular lens (IOL) opacification had been shortlisted for the award. As I sat in the auditorium, nervous and excited to know who would get the prize, visuals of my life flashed before my eyes—the prolonged struggle against poverty and dodging life's every curveball to finally reach here.

Thomas A. Weingeist, PhD, MD and president of AAO, made the announcement: 'The American Academy of Ophthalmology is pleased to present the Best of the Show Video award to Dr Suresh K. Pandey.' I got up, squared my shoulders, and walked up to the stage feeling a deep sense of gratitude for my parents, grandfather, teachers and everyone who inspired me on my journey as an ophthalmologist—most importantly, my spiritual gurus, Pandit Shri Ram Sharma Acharya and Vandniya Mataji, without whose guidance and blessings my life would be incomplete.

The next year, at the 2003 meeting of the AAO, held at Anaheim, CA, USA, I was honoured with an AAO Achievement Award. At thirty-five, I was perhaps the youngest Indian ophthalmologist to have received this honour. It was presented to me by Michael R. Redmond, MD, then president of AAO. During my five-year stay in the USA, I was fortunate to receive several prestigious awards from the American Society of Cataract and Refractive Surgery (ASCRS), the European Society of Cataract and Refractive Surgery (ESCRS), and, of course, the AAO, for presenting the best paper of the session, best video and best posters. I was lucky to get international recognition after the ASCRS and ESCRS Film Festival Awards (known as the 'Oscars of Ophthalmology'). During these award ceremonies, I walked with pride not just because I was happy for myself but because I was a representative of my country—a land known for the hard work and determination of its people.

After completing my MS in Ophthalmology, I joined Storm Eye Institute, Medical University of South Carolina, Charleston, SC, USA in July 1998. Once I had finished my anterior segment fellowship there, I joined John A. Moran Eye Center, University of Utah, USA as an instructor in June 2002. I was living in the USA for seven years. One day, I suddenly became aware of the fact that my life abroad had served its purpose. It was now time to return to my motherland to be of service to the millions who lived with curable blindness. I moved back to India in December 2005 and established an ophthalmology practice built on ethics and empathy, in Kota. The new city opened us up to a large family of the scores of coaching students who came to attend coaching to clear entrance exams and build their futures. When my wife Dr Vidushi and I interacted with them, we were often asked about our failures and the challenges we faced to reach where we are today. Their questions steered me towards memory lane—for the first time in a long time, I thought about how I reached where I was.

How did a left-handed eye surgeon successfully perform over one lakh eye surgeries? A desire then began to grip me—a desire to tell my story; to pick apart my life and unravel its many threads; to chronicle and reflect upon the fifty-five years' journey from an impoverished village to the global stage. My motive in telling my story is to inspire and encourage my readers—to give you a pat on your back, a gentle nudge and tender motivation to follow your dreams. Because if I can, you can, too.

# 1

# Pandemic, Pain, Profession and Prayers

## My Journey to the Inner self

*Picture Abhi Baki Hai, The Show Must Go On . . .*

This was the message of Padma Shri awardee, Dr K.K. Agarwal, in one of his last educational videos about COVID-19 in May 2021, before he added that he too had been afflicted by the coronavirus. In his video, Dr Agarwal mentioned, 'I have COVID-19 pneumonia, which is progressive. But even then, remember Raj Kapoor's words "the show must go on".' He passed away on 17 May 2021 at Delhi's All India Institute of Medical Sciences (AIIMS) after a long battle with COVID-19. The sixty-two-year-old was a cardiologist, head of the Heart Care Foundation of India (HCFI) and former president of the Indian Medical Association (IMA). He had received the Dr B.C. Roy Award in 2005 and the Padma Shri in 2010.

The entire medical fraternity as well as the public mourned the demise of Dr Agarwal and thousands of other COVID-19 warriors. I was discussing Dr Agarwal with his classmate Dr Akhil Saxena (son of Dr M.R. Saxena, Kota) and his wife Dr Nikita Saxena, when he came to me for his cataract surgery in June 2021. Dr Agarwal and Dr

Saxena had completed MBBS, from the Mahatma Gandhi Institute of Medical Sciences, Wardha in 1983. Dr Saxena was a hostel roommate of his during their MBBS days. He was remembering his friend Kishan, fondly called 'Kissu' by his friends, who was eccentric and very knowledgeable—he used to keep all his books on his bed and slept on the floor himself.

I also got an opportunity to meet Dr K.K. Agarwal when he was the president of the Indian Medical Association. He felicitated me at AIIMS, New Delhi on 7 January 2017 with the IMA Community Service Award. Dr K.K. Agrawal had also paid a visit to Kota and Dr Akhil Saxena, Dr Nikita Saxena and other members of the IMA Kota branch were all very sad to know the news of his passing during the second wave of the COVID-19 pandemic.

## 'Quarantine', 'Outbreak' and 'Pandemic'

It was about thirty-four years ago that I first learned the words 'quarantine', 'outbreak' and 'pandemic' as part of preventive and social medicine (PSM) during my second year of MBBS curriculum. Years later, these words were splashed all across the media, hoardings and on the lips of the public. Government authorities were trying their best to curtail the COVID-19 pandemic with doctors and healthcare workers on the frontline as corona warriors. The government machinery was very serious about dealing effectively with COVID-19 which had been declared as a global pandemic on 11 March 2020. Although social distancing is the most effective way to contain the spread of the virus, it is not easy to implement for healthcare professionals, who were required to maintain direct contact with COVID-19 patients, putting them at very high risk of being infected. Frontline healthcare professionals were particularly vulnerable, owing to their commitment to contain the disease. The World Health Organization (WHO) estimates that between 80,000 and 1,80,000 healthcare workers may have died from COVID-19 in the period between January 2020 and January 2023, of about 6,722,949 deaths.

On the evening of 24 March 2020, the Government of India under Prime Minister Narendra Modi, ordered a nationwide lockdown for twenty-one days, limiting the movement of the entire 138 crore population of India as a preventive measure against the COVID-19 pandemic. At the time, just a few cases of COVID-19 had been reported in Rajasthan—a group of Italian tourists. A hospital in Bhilwara (Rajasthan) had also operated upon a COVID-19 positive patient, resulting in the transmission of the infection to their doctors and staff. This news was published on the front pages of newspapers in the local/national media and shown on news channels across the country. The media trial began and the hospital and its doctors were labelled as 'super spreaders' of COVID-19. There were several incidences of violence against doctors as well. Besides physiological threats, such a public health emergency affected the psyche of healthcare workers (HCWs), including work stress, fear of infection and helplessness. To add to this, several messages started circulating on social media defaming doctors and hospitals, who were fighting against the pandemic on the frontlines. Government hospitals stopped examining routine cases, as well as offering emergency services in view of the need to get all doctors and staff members to focus on COVID-19 cases. This was during the first wave of COVID-19 and there were still a lot of myths about transmission in the public forum. Every day, some new guidelines were issued and no one was sure about the line of treatment or how to manage the complications.

We closed the operation theatre (OT) of SuVi Eye Institute & Lasik Laser Centre, Kota, on 24 March 2020, for routine eye surgeries. We also implemented all safety measures and started attending only to emergency cases. We read with sorrow the sad news of the death of Dr Li Wenliang, the Chinese ophthalmologist and whistleblower, who alerted the local authorities in Wuhan about the COVID-19 pneumonia.[*] We sent around messages and put up signages to tell patients to avoid coming to the hospital unless it was an emergency, and remained available for WhatsApp or online consultation.

## Panic, Pain and the Power of Prayers

During the initial months of the pandemic, I was staying on the third floor of SuVi Eye Hospital with my seventy-eight-year-old mother, medico wife and fourteen-year-old daughter. I was hesitant to spend time with my daughter for several months for fear of transmission. Every day, I was seeing needy patients who came to me with great hope. My team and I provided free online consultation to more than 10,000 patients during the pandemic. We took great care of our team by following all the safety measures and precautions to safeguard them.

During the lockdown, at about 5 P.M. on 19 April 2020, we got a call from Bhilwara. A three-year-old girl, Yashasvi Gupta, had injured her right eye badly with a knife. She needed emergency eye surgery not only to preserve her eyesight but also to conserve the shape of the globe (eyeball). Most eye surgeons (in government and private setups) had explicitly refused to take on her case due to the media trial of the Bhilwara Hospital.[†] Routine surgeries at the government hospital were closed as all resources had been focused on dealing with the pandemic. Secondly, her surgery needed to be performed under general anaesthesia. Most of the anaesthetics refused to give the intubation anaesthesia as there were chances of

---

[*] 'Li Wenliang: Coronavirus kills Chinese whistleblower doctor', BBC, 7 February 2020. Available at: https://www.bbc.com/news/world-asia-china-51403795.

[†] Rohit Parihar, 'How Bhilwara became the Epicentre of the Covid-19 outbreak', India Today Insight, 29 March 2020. Available at: https://www.indiatoday.in/web-exclusive/story/how-bhilwara-became-the-epicentre-of-the-covid-19-outbreak-1661098-2020-03-29.

COVID-19 transmission while intubating the child or putting the tube in the throat. The girl's parents contacted at least twelve eye doctors and various hospitals, but failed to get any help. We also expressed our inability to help them as our anaesthetists were not available. After four hours, they called us again and started crying, pleading us to help them save the eye of their only child.

I could not sleep the entire night and kept praying for the child. In the morning, Dr Vidushi and I decided to perform the eye surgery. We requested Dr Vijay Goyal to give general anaesthesia. He agreed, after ensuring that all precautions had been taken. The surgery took two and a half hours as it was really a large corneo-scleral perforation with irido-dialysis (iris tear). Dr Vidushi did the repair of the cornea, sclera and the iris.

The surgery was successful. Yashasvi recovered well and was discharged after twenty-four hours. When I examined her, she was able to count her fingers. Upon seeing this, her parents' faces were drenched in tears—tears of happiness at their prayers having been answered. Later, Yashasvi underwent a second surgery that removed a cataract and implanted an intraocular lens in her right eye. A third surgery was performed to clear the membrane from its visual axis. Today, the child has regained almost normal vision. We managed at least twelve such cases during the COVID-19 era and every case was both difficult and unique. We did not close our doors even for a day and our emergency eye services continued for the needy. Looking back, I feel that this was nothing short of a miracle and we were driven, perhaps, by the power of prayers, conscience and positivity.

## My Journey to the Inner Self

As I was reading about the news of thousands of doctors and healthcare workers sacrificing their lives while fighting against COVID-19, the negative media coverage and social media posts forced me to introspect. I thought about the medical profession in general and my own medical journey in particular. Despite all the negativity around doctors and the burgeoning pressure mounting on them, we felt like a community during the raging pandemic and I tried to recall why I had always wanted to become a doctor.

I travelled down the memory lane to reminisce about life's innumerable challenges that I had had to battle to get to where I am today. I also regularly received news of a few of my colleagues who were infected and admitted to the hospital and recovered, while a few others sadly passed away either due to COVID-19 itself or related complications. I was very sad to hear of the passing of countless other people globally, including several friends, relatives and the renowned duo: Dr K.K. Agarwal and Dr Ashok Panagariya. They visited Kota upon my invitation and participated in health awareness events while I was working as Secretary of IMA, Kota.

Distressing news of the death of doctors, friends and some of my patients during the second deadly wave of COVID-19 motivated me to prepare my own will and this memoir in order to share my journey, with an intention to motivate readers and medical professionals.

I am in no way specially qualified to write this autobiography for I am neither a celebrity doctor, nor have I accomplished anything spectacular, except for the fact I was born in a village, worked hard at my studies and was able to become an eye surgeon who has successfully performed more than one lakh eye surgeries in his career and touched many lives. I am sharing my life story of having made it to this juncture against all odds.

This is my story . . .

# 2

# Dadaji

## My Earliest Hero

*'The greatest thing in the world is not so much where we are, but in what direction we are moving.'*

—Oliver Wendell Holmes

There was a great din at school. The students were chatting and laughing when the Block Development Officer (BDO) and the local *pradhan*\* walked in for a surprise inspection. He eyed the class intently and asked in his gruff voice, 'Is there anyone who wants to volunteer to give a speech?' The students grew nervous. They shifted uncomfortably on their benches. No one wanted to volunteer. I raised my hand. The BDO nodded and invited me to speak on any topic of my choice.

I wracked my brain for something I may have read and immediately began narrating the story of a famous space scientist, Dr A.P.J. Abdul Kalam, that I had read in the *Junior Science Digest*. 'A dream is not what you see while you are asleep, a dream is something

---

\* A gram pradhan or *mukhiya* is a decision-maker, elected by the village-level constitutional body of local self-government called the Gram Sabha (village government) in India.

7

that does not let you sleep,' I repeated his famous words. The BDO, pradhan and our teachers were astonished. 'What is your dream?' the pradhan asked me. 'What do you want to become in the future?'

'An eye doctor,' I answered with a glint in my eye.

## God of the Sick Children

It was the year 1968. As soon as I was born a little before the eighth month of pregnancy had ended, I contracted neonatal jaundice. I was weak and sickly, suffered from frequent vomiting, diarrhoea and respiratory infections, and would later on be told that I had a ventricular septal defect or a small hole in my heart. My parents admitted me to J.K. Lon Hospital in Kota, Rajasthan, where my condition deteriorated further due to septicaemia, a blood infection. The doctors were close to giving up on me and said the chances of survival were thin. But my mother did not lose hope. We were strapped for resources, barely making ends meet—the only way my mother could afford my treatment was by selling her ornaments. So that's what she did to buy me more time. Now my fate was in the hands of Dr M.R. Saxena, a famous paediatrician of Kota, who was often called the 'God of ill children'. Dr Saxena treated me for almost a month and saved my life. The day I was declared safe, my parents started dreaming that I would become a miracle-making doctor like Dr Saxena. I was on the edge and my parents realized then—as I do today—that there's nothing more valuable than one's health. When you are ill or injured, your normal way of life is disrupted. Doctors have the incredible opportunity to help you restore your life to normalcy and even save you from death itself.

## Ballia, Bhiwani and My Beautiful Village

I went back home to a village called Mohna, a beautiful place surrounded by mountains and seasonal waterfalls, thick forests brimming with wildlife, situated in the Rawatbhata tahsil Chittorgarh district in Rajasthan. Our village is about 800 years old; it was a revenue collection centre of the Udaipur princely state that fell under the Bhainsrodgarh base. A ginning factory, oil mill and cotton mill were established in this village by Bhainsrodgarh Thikanedar, Rawat Himmat Singh Chundawat. There were three big step-wells, temples and several wells for the storage of grains and to be used as stables for horses, which are still there. Before Independence, there was a police station in Mohna village, which was later moved to Gandhisagar after 1947, when Gandhisagar was still a part of Rajasthan.

My father, Late Shri Kameshwar Prasad Pandey, was a respected school teacher in that village and other adjoining villages. My mother, Smt. Maya Devi Pandey, was a homemaker and played the most vital role in building my character by teaching me the values of life. For my parents, the priority was to make their four children into good human beings, above all else. They believed education is the 'best tool' to counter ignorance, poverty and also enhance one's self-worth. But the adult who led by example and exhibited the most humanity, inspiring me every day, was my grandfather, Late Dr Kamta Prasad Pandey.

My grandfather was born on 24 February 1916 in a village called Pura, Ballia district, Uttar Pradesh. He was a freedom fighter who migrated from Ballia to Rajasthan during the Baghi Ballia (Rebel Ballia) movement in 1944. He participated in India's freedom movement and was imprisoned along with freedom fighter Late Shri Cheetu Pandey (known as Tiger of Ballia). He was trained at Kishan Lal Jalan Eye Hospital in Bhiwani, Haryana, during 1937–38. There, he learnt the art of cataract surgery and other techniques for treating various eye-related ailments. In those days, he was one of the few doctors who knew the technique of intracapsular cataract surgery, also known as large incision cataract surgery.[*]

---

[*] Intracapsular cataract extraction (ICCE) involves the removal of the crystalline lens and the surrounding lens capsule in one piece.

When I was a child, I recall that I used to play with thick aphakic glasses that my grandfather had in his clinic. Aphakic glasses are plus 10 dioptre thick glasses that were used to correct vision six weeks after cataract surgery during the decade of 1970–80, when artificial (intraocular) lens implantation was not done. I recall when we would put on the aphakic glasses, everything would look magnified. From the age of five, I noticed a long line of patients in front of our old house since the crack of dawn. A few children of my age would lead their grandparents by the hand, who were unable to see anything due to mature cataracts. Dadaji would start seeing patients early in the morning and would see more than 100 people in a day. He did not charge any fees. Most of the patients were villagers and would bring grains, vegetables, milk, ghee, etc. as a token of respect for my grandfather. He was completely dedicated to eliminating their suffering. Even though he was an eye specialist, he would treat other common ailments too.

Dadaji always told me that he felt blessed as God had given him an opportunity to serve as a healer. 'I am very fortunate that by God's grace, I'm able to relieve so many patients of their pain,' he said. He taught me the five Cs for becoming a good healer—compassion, competence, confidence, conscience and commitment. Even after forty three years, his teachings are ingrained in my mind.

## Cataract—Commonest Cause of Blindness

Cataract, also known as *motiyabind* in Hindi, remains the most common cause of blindness in the elderly population globally. Age-related cataract is very common among the elderly in villages due to their exposure to ultraviolet light and poor nutrition. Some patients develop mature cataracts even before they turn fifty. Until the 1980s, cataract surgery wasn't advanced. It used a large, almost 12 mm incision, lasted ten minutes, and the patients were required to wear thick—plus 10 dioptre—glasses after surgery. Intraocular lens (or artificial lens) implantation had not yet started in India and the surgery could only be performed when the cataract was completely mature.

Patients came to my grandfather with mature cataracts in both eyes and poor vision. In 1980, one of his patients was my school headmaster's mother. She had lost her vision due to age-related cataract and had fallen down in her house and injured herself. But she was terrified of the word 'surgery'. Due to this fear, she refused to get operated upon or even consult a doctor despite her condition. When my headmaster mentioned this incident, I decided to take matters into my own hands. I—a twelve-year-old boy—went to his house and reassured his mother that she would not feel any pain or discomfort. She agreed. The next day, Dadaji operated on her and she regained her vision in a few days.

Since that day, my teachers began to introduce me as 'the eye doctor's grandson'. They finally understood the inspiration behind my dream to become an ophthalmologist. I was glad. Nothing made me happier than to be known by my Dadaji's name. Every day, the respect they bestowed upon him moved and spurred me on to a career in medicine. If I had any doubts, conversations with my grandfather would help reinforce the desire.

## Nationalism and The 'Nagwa' Connection

My Dadima, Late Smt. Ram Shringari Devi, was born in Nagwa (Ballia) on 9 March 1917 in the same village as Mangal Pandey, who is widely regarded as the first martyr in India's First War of Independence in 1857.* I was brought up listening to the stories of atrocities of the soldiers against freedom fighters, when India was

---

* Mangal Pandey (19 July 1827, Nagwa – 8 April 1857, Barrackpore) was an Indian soldier who led the attack on British officers on 29 March 1857—the first major incident of what came to be known as the Indian or Sepoy Mutiny. In India, the uprising is often called the First War of Independence or by other similar names.

under British rule. My grandparents and parents emphasized family values and the importance of *rashtradharma* and *rashtra bhakti* to help us respectfully maintain the freedom that had come after a lot of sacrifices. These stories instilled deep moral values in my mind which propelled Dr Vidushi and I to return to serve in India in 2005, from Sydney, Australia. We watched the movie *Mangal Pandey: The Rising* on my birthday in August 2005 in Sydney. As we sat watching, the entire recollection of the many stories of Mangal Pandey narrated by my grandparents and my visit to Dadaji's village, Nagwa, flashed in my mind.

One day, my Dadima asked me to convince Dadaji to accompany her on the Char Dham Yatra, the Hindu pilgrimage. When Dadaji returned from an eye camp, I sat with him and struck up a conversation. 'Dadaji, why don't you take a break and join Dadima on the pilgrimage?' I asked.

My grandfather laughed. 'But, I am on a pilgrimage right now,' he said.

I was stumped. 'How?' I asked.

'I give sight to the blind and help them see the world—*Tamso Ma Jyotirgamaya*, which means "from darkness lead me to the light". God has given me this very important task to help the blind move from darkness to light and make a difference in their lives. This is my pilgrimage.'

I was startled at his words—words that I remember to this day.

Dadaji practised what he preached every day of his life. He would spend the first three weeks each month travelling and conducting eye camps across Rajasthan, Uttar Pradesh and Madhya Pradesh. Only during the last week of every month did he stay with us at Mohna. When he came home, so did his patients. A serpentine queue of the visually impaired would gather outside our home. I would wake up and see patients and their relatives thronging, waiting for hours to meet him. Dadaji was known for his perennial availability and a kind-hearted approach towards his patients. When these patients would regain their lost eyesight, their gratitude would know no bounds. They would approach him with folded hands and fall at his feet. He was almost like God for them. They would regard him as the saviour of their vision. It was heartwarming to see them express their gratitude towards my grandfather.

The more I watched Dadaji at work, the more my desire to become an ophthalmologist strengthened. Like him, I wanted to help patients regain their eyesight so that they could lead better lives. But like me, this desire had also burned in my father's heart. He too had wanted to become a doctor, but a variety of challenges had kept his dream unfulfilled. Through me, my father hoped to fulfil his dream. But there I had many obstacles of my own to conquer.

## Overcoming Obstacles with a Never-Say-Die Attitude

They began with the quality of my life at home. Ours was a joint family where issues that affected one member were felt by the others. Dadima grappled with a highly introverted personality, and we suspected that my father, too, had inherited the same condition. This mental turmoil affected his government job and prevented him from giving us the paternal care and emotional support that we needed during our early childhood. He spent most of his time reading books in his room. He rarely stepped out and hence missed attending many family functions, including birthdays and weddings.

But I had an affectionate relationship with my father. He believed that I was his most obedient son so he often involved me in his adventures. One day, I joined him in his experiment to turn common metal into gold. I knew it wouldn't work but I humoured him. Others in the family, however, were not as patient. Some of our relatives revolted against his behaviour. Dadima protected him fiercely, but when she passed away, the overall situation worsened. When my grandfather wrote his will, he excluded my family and the house we lived in. My father moved court against Dadaji.

On the one hand was the growing acrimony in the family, disputes that soured the home environment; and on the other were everyday routine tasks like going to school barefooted and coming back home to study under a lantern.

I shall elaborate. I clearly remember the year 1977 (towards the end of the Emergency declared by Prime Minister Indra Gandhi) when I was nine years old. The nation faced a tough time and so did my parents. Our family was a joint family with my grandfather, grandmother, uncle, two of my aunts, and my father. Everything was going well till late 1976. After the death of my grandmother, the situation started changing and we noticed a sudden change in behaviour of our close family members turning from a happy to a hostile environment. My father missed attending the wedding of one of our close relatives in Ballia, UP, one summer, since it was planned at short notice. This further strained the relationship between the brothers and their father, and culminated in long disputes over ancestral property.

My grandmother had always supported my father and his family, but sadly, she passed away on 20 February 1977. After her death, the situation quickly worsened. My parents were greatly distressed at the growing hostility at home and decided to move away in order to ensure we all had the peace of mind we required, especially since I was a young, impressionable school-going child.

My father purchased a small piece of land from Panchayat Samiti in Mohna during an auction and also contributed financially towards the construction of a new, four-bedroom house. However, after the death of my grandmother, my father was compelled to leave. We left the newly constructed family home to live in an old, one-room house which was very small for our family of six. On most nights, either my sister or I had to sleep under the bed. It was the most difficult, depressing, and dark phase of my life when as an eleven-year-old boy, I was experiencing such challenging difficulties and heartache.

* * *

Our village was supplied with electricity in late 1985, but we (my three siblings and I) still had to use a lantern to study. The electricity supply to our house came through the new family home and was disconnected almost every day by one of our hostile family members a few hours after dusk to annoy us and disturb our study.

Between 1977–80, my mother's health had also started declining. My elder sister Usha Pandey and I started cooking for our family as my mother became confined to her bed due to asthma, heavy menstrual bleeding and extreme weakness. We visited the local doctor and he referred my mother to M.B.S. Hospital in Kota. My mother was admitted there and a blood transfusion was done. After a complete check-up, the cause of her weakness was pinned down—a fibroid of the uterus resulting in dysfunctional intrauterine bleeding which had caused her haemoglobin level to fall to 7 grams per decilitre. The doctors suggested surgery to remove the uterine fibroid but the procedure was delayed due to low haemoglobin and her asthma.

As would now have become apparent, my early life was ridden with several problems and obstacles. This time in my life felt like a long never-ending *Amavasya* or new moon night. All of these events were enough to disrupt my study schedule, completely shatter my self-confidence and push anyone over the edge into depression.

But I always had a never-say-die attitude. I was desperate to get rid of the negativity and misery that surrounded me and began to take solace in my studies. I almost grew addicted to studying. There were times when I was overwhelmed by our financial and familial crises and found it impossible to focus. There were times when I was almost weighed down with depression. Sometimes, I would worry that like everyone else in the village, I too was fated to live a mundane life, merely living from paycheck to paycheck. There were times when I thought that it was pointless to fight against the odds—perhaps my destiny *was* to spend my entire life in that tiny village.

No matter what happened, my mother was firmly on my side, loving and supporting me throughout my life. Of the four of us siblings, I was the most obedient. One day, my father scolded me for taking a book of his without his permission. He was a passionate reader and intolerant of anyone intruding upon him. But my mother intervened, reprimanding him for screaming at me. 'You should not have scolded him for reading your book,' she said. But our family troubles didn't end at mundane quarrels. Eventually, due to genetic predisposition and the disturbed family atmosphere, one of our close family members developed an unknown psychiatric condition.

He was very intelligent in his childhood with outstanding memory. He could recall any address, phone number or details he read in a book or any past incident. At the age of fourteen, we noticed changes in his memory, intelligence and behaviour. He developed unusual fear, started hearing voices, getting paranoid that someone was following him and was after his life. Similar details were also communicated to us by his school teachers. All of us tried to counsel him but his problem only deteriorated. Finally, we decided to consult a doctor. My mother and I took him to a psychiatrist in Kota. To our shock, the diagnosis was paranoid schizophrenia. 'The exact causes of schizophrenia are unknown. Research suggests a combination of physical, genetic, psychological and environmental factors can make it more likely for a person to develop the condition. Some people may be prone to schizophrenia and a stressful or emotional life event might trigger a psychotic episode,' the psychiatrist informed my mother. This was a matter of great concern.

I, too, began to grow worried that I might be afflicted with psychiatric illness. There were many reasons to justify my concern as it ran in our family—my grandmother and my father also suffered from some psychiatric issue, although because they never visited a doctor, a formal diagnosis was never made.

* * *

Contrary to Dadaji's outgoing personality and larger-than-life image, my father believed in very simple living. He always held a grudge against his father as he too had wanted to become a doctor but had never got his encouragement and support. However, my father taught us that education is the best tool to overcome adversities like poverty. Babuji focussed on providing a good education to his four children. He would save each and every penny to support our education. He appreciated Mahatma Gandhi for his simple living, and was also influenced by Pandit Shri Ram Sharma Acharya, Ram Charan Mahendra, etc. who advised against wasteful expenditure or *fizool kharchi*.

My sister Smt. Usha Pandey and I moved to Rawatbhata for our education in 1982. We stayed in a rented room and fended for ourselves. I had only one set of uniform—a white shirt and khaki pant—which I would wear to school daily. I later arranged for one more shirt that I would wear on Thursdays, when we were mandated to wear clothes other than our uniform. Many of my classmates mocked me for this. However, I told them that I washed my uniform on Sunday and if I had no problem with having only one set, they should not either. When my teachers and classmates met my father during his visit to the school, they were surprised at his simplicity. However, a few fellow students relentlessly made fun of me. It was obvious that they were jealous of my academic performance and wanted to pull me down with their negative comments. I started developing an inferiority complex due to my family problems, financial constraints and repeated teasing by my classmates. I was depressed for quite a few weeks.

However, I quickly overcame this phase of depression by reading the great inspirational stories of the former Indian Prime Minister Lal Bahadur Shastri, and freedom fighter and spiritual guru, Pandit Shri Ram Sharma Acharya. I could correlate everything with their teachings, but it took me a few years to rid myself of the inferiority complex.

Being raised in a family suffering from psychiatric illness carried a lot of challenges and difficulties due to poor self-esteem, negativity and of course, depression. I had experienced the hardship very closely during my childhood. While writing these lines, the entire scene is moving in my mind like a film—how I faced the atrocities, insults, from 1977 to 1980 and how I was very angry and wanted to take revenge on everyone involved. I channelled all those negative emotions into striving to become somebody from nobody. I read inspirational books and motivational stories, and fought very hard to overcome all the challenges and difficulties. I was far too determined to overcome all adversities by becoming an eye doctor, support my parents and family, and also to get my relative the best psychiatric help money could buy, to be bogged down. I worked very hard at my studies.

Supporting my family taught me how to be patient, passionate and persistent. It also made me resilient. I learnt how to face adversities with optimism. With the support of my mother at each and every step, and using my Dadaji as inspiration, I refused to let my problems get in my way and diligently fought against all distractions to focus on my studies.

But there was little I could do about our financial situation, which was often the subject of ridicule at home. If any of us fell ill, my mother would have to take us to Kota as there were no medical facilities in our village. She would walk for two kilometers to get the bus to Rawatbhata and then get another bus to reach Kota. There, our relatives would help us and also accompany my mother to visit the doctors. However, they would make fun of my mother's simple attire, our rural roots and ways. They would sarcastically call her 'foreign wali masi' (foreigner aunt). Initially perturbed, I learned eventually to take such jokes in my stride and respond to them solely by becoming someone significant in my life. My passion and determination to support my parents became strong. Now when I look back, I also understand that my parents were constrained in multiple ways, both emotionally and financially. Despite that, they did what they could for me and my three siblings. As I grew older, I realized that it was upon me to transform my life and the life of my parents.

## The Light at the End of the Tunnel

In 1982, when I was fourteen years old, I got a golden opportunity. I had scored 88 per cent in my senior secondary school exams and topped the entire Chittorgarh district. It was a watershed moment for me as those marks meant that I had qualified for the National Talent Search Examination (NTSE) scholarship for further studies. The scholarship offered me a princely sum of ₹5,100. But, more importantly, it acted as a tremendous morale booster for me. I already had the determination, the only thing dampening my spirit was my finances. But now with the scholarship, there was no looking back.

In August 1981, my grandfather suffered from a heart attack and was admitted to M.B.S. hospital in Kota under the supervision of Dr A.Q. Khan and Dr K.K. Pareek. He passed away on 16 September 1981. I visited him and had the opportunity to talk to him a few times. A few days before he passed away, I visited him and touched his feet. He affectionately put his palm on my head and blessed me. 'Respected Dadaji,' I said, 'I also want to give the gift of sight to patients and follow in your footsteps'. In that moment, despite his illness, I thought he beamed and forgot all about his struggles for a brief second.

Forty-four years later, while writing these lines, I do not have any ill feelings for any one for their deeds. I have released all my negativity and replaced it with positivity. I worked hard and thanked life for the opportunities that made me into a stronger and more resilient person. I thank God for giving me a tough time, otherwise I may not have tried hard enough. I now deliberately go about my everyday life with plenty of positivity—I am happier, healthier, handle stress better, and get along well with others.

# 3

# Early Whiff of Success

## Entering Medical College

*'Motivation is like food for the brain. You cannot get enough in one sitting. It needs continual and regular top-ups.'*

—Peter Davies

My grandfather took out a plastic box containing the von Graefe knife[*] from his lab coat pocket. The knife glinted in the morning sunlight. 'The von Graefe knife,' I said. After sterilization of all the surgical instruments, he cleaned the left eye and periocular area with spirit and anesthetized the eye by injecting lignocaine (an anesthetic solution) using a long needle attached to a glass syringe. He then covered it with sterile green linen and used an eye speculum to open the left eye. He entered in the left eye from 3 o'clock and came out at 9 o'clock and created a large 12 mm corneal incision. He then used his forceps to remove the cataract. I watched in awe as not even a drop of blood was spilled. How quick and elegant! I was

---

[*] The von Graefe knife is a specialized knife for cataract surgery which was designed by a German ophthalmologist, Dr Albrecht von Graefe (22 May 1828–20 July 1870).

dumbfounded. 'Bravo!' I said again and again till I woke up. It was a dream. I sat up and was still reflecting on the made-up surgery when I saw that a few people had gathered outside our house. My packed bag lay in a corner of the living room. I asked my mother about the crowd. 'They are here for you,' she said. I couldn't believe what I had heard.

## Scholarship, Summer Vacation and Studies

The news of my scholarship had spread like wildfire. Several families in the village had arrived to congratulate me. For the first time in my life, there was a crowd thronging outside my house not for Dadaji, but me. Shortly after, I bid my family a teary goodbye and left for my new school in Rawatbhata, a town famous for its atomic energy power plant. A completely new life was waiting there for me. Every day, I would wake up early to study, cook my meal on a *sigri*, go to school, and return to cook and study before I slept. I was only fourteen but proved adept at housekeeping and cooking. The pre-medical tests (PMT) were still three years away, but I was dreaming about excelling in it and starting my career as a doctor.

During summer vacations, I would visit Kota and accompany my elder sister to her examination at Janki Devi Bajaj (JDB) Government Girls' College, Kota. We would stay at 'Sunder Dharmshala', where room number 6 was given to us free of cost and all the Kanyakubja Brahmins. My sister would study for her B.A. exams and I would accompany her to the examination centre. I would borrow books for the next class and study them during the summer vacation. I would finish my entire biology, some parts of chemistry, and physics during the summer time. During one of the summer vacations, I visited my maternal uncle, Advocate Anand Ballabh Tiwari, in Kanpur, where I urged my cousins to take me to the Late Ganesh Shankar Vidyarthi Medical College nearby. It was an odd getaway choice for any teenager and my cousins didn't hesitate in pointing this out.

I didn't listen. I wanted to go to the medical college and sneak a peek into the anatomy dissection hall, the physiology and pathology laboratories. If children my age in cities had posters of their favourite sportspersons and movie stars on the walls of their rooms, I had the poster of a human body and skeleton, using my savings.

Becoming a doctor meant everything to me. Dr Joseph Murphy wrote in his book *Believe in Yourself*: 'People who are low in confidence, need a direction in life or a guiding light to keep them motivated'. I was deeply in awe of doctors and the power they wielded. I wanted to be a leader in healthcare and have the final say on treatment decisions so I could help improve patients' lives. I had observed that when doctors talked, people usually listened. Even outside the work setting, doctors are regarded highly. That's what I wanted for myself.

In 1983, after I completed my eleventh grade from Rawatbhata, I moved to the Government College in Rampura (MP), where Dadaji's friend, Dr Ram Pratap Gupta, worked as a professor. Here, I completed BSc Part I and ranked first at Vikram University, Ujjain, MP. This is also when I started preparing for the PMT. My friends, Kamlesh Chandel, Man Singh Chandel and Jai Prakash Singh, Somesh Gupta, lived nearby and I would often go to their house at Nani Choti (Chandrawat Palace) during the weekends at 9 P.M. to study till dawn. Coaching for PMT was not available that time. Thanks to this study group, group discussions, rapid-fire question and answer sessions, I cleared the PMT on my first attempt and was selected for admission in the Government Medical College at Jabalpur, later known as the Netaji Subhash Chandra Bose Medical College.

When I look back, I realize that my strong inclination to read and write helped me excel academically. At school, I was the student who couldn't even dream of disobeying the teacher. This was because my parents taught me that education is the 'best weapon' to counter ignorance, poverty and enhance one's self-worth. Once I had qualified the for entrance, I felt grateful for these early experiences. But before I took admission into medical college, there was something essential I had to do.

* * *

For many years, I had heard stories about how Dr M.R. Saxena had saved my life and now, with a promising medical career ahead of me, I decided to pay him a visit. My father and I went to his clinic. Dr Saxena was hard at work. On any given day, he would treat about 100 ailing children. When Dr Saxena saw us, he called us in. My father whispered into my ear to touch his feet. I immediately did so. 'Congratulations, Suresh,' Dr Saxena said. 'But remember that the journey to become a caring doctor who fulfils patient expectations is not at all easy,' he cautioned. 'As a paediatrician, I have the responsibility of looking after children who come to me in pain. Seeing them smile after the treatment is just so rewarding. Seeing their parents and grandparents heave a sigh of relief when they get better gives me pure joy. The patient comes to me with 100 per cent trust and faith, and I do my best to solve their problems,' he explained.

'What is the most difficult part, doctor?' I asked.

'Balance,' Dr Saxena said. 'You need to master the art of balancing your personal and professional life. People place their expectations in doctors without realizing that we are not God. We are humans who are simply putting our knowledge together to do our best.'

Dr Saxena's words were as enlightening for a starry-eyed medical student then, as they are today.

## Step by Step: My Journey as a Medical Student

My life's dream was finally close to being fulfilled. On 5 November 1986, my father and I reached Jabalpur, a beautiful city situated on the banks of the Narmada River in Madhya Pradesh. I had received a letter of admission from Government Medical College, Jabalpur. A new chapter of life, brimming with new opportunities as well as new challenges, had begun.

140 students filled the classroom. Their eyes were glued to a green board covered with details about the syllabi and timelines. I slunk in like a cat, unsure of my place in the lecture hall, in the medical college and perhaps, in the world. The previous day, I had stood by the auditorium staircase and watched my parents walk away till they had disappeared from sight. The first year students' orientation had just finished and my parents were returning home. I waved at them vigorously for what felt like several minutes as hot tears rolled down my cheeks.

Afterwards, I left for my room—a stone's throw from the campus. During the first month, sometimes the seniors would ask all juniors to gather and introduce themselves at the hostel while singing, dancing, sharing jokes, etc. I decided to face the situation wisely and tried to enjoy the process as much as possible. As a result, I became very popular among the seniors and they extended all sorts of help to me. The forced interaction with them contributed tremendously in the conversion of my shy self into a confident, thick-skinned individual, ready to face all the challenges and adversities of my professional and personal life.

In the anatomy lecture, one day, I claimed a spot at the back. All my life, I had been a front-bencher—the zealous student with a spring in his arm. But that day, I did not want to be observed. However, Professor T.M. Garg (the head of the anatomy department) caught sight of me anyway. 'Hey, blue shirt,' he called. I was terrified. Seniors had told me how strict the anatomy teachers were. It was not uncommon for them to punish first-year medical students by making them stand facing the green board for sixty minutes. And this was the head of the department! I stood up. He asked me my name and where I hailed from. His long, greasy hair was tied at the back and his forehead was smeared with three horizontal lines of *vibhuti* (holy ash), with a red dot of *kumkum* in the middle. 'Come and sit in the front,' he ordered. There was pin-drop silence in the class, students looking from me to him. I did as I was told, and just like that, my nervousness dissipated a bit. I felt recognized.

A few days later, Professor Garg, Dr S.K. Verma Sr, Dr V. Malviya, Dr S.K. Shrivastava, Dr S.K. Verma Jr, Dr B.K. Guha, Dr A. Dixit, Dr P.C. Jain marched us to the dissection lab, where a clever signboard greeted us. 'This is the only place where the dead teach the living. Respect it and maintain silence.' I read the board and smiled. I had begun to adjust to my new life. Introduction rituals, singing and dancing together with our seniors had been routine at the hostel and they had driven all the fear out of me. I was eager to learn in class. I was in shock when I entered the vast anatomy dissection hall. On the tables were treated corpses, the dead bodies. The hall reeked of formalin, a chemical used to preserve cadavers. In the late 1980s, this and other preservatives were injected into the blood vessels immediately after death so that the corpse would not decompose and remain in normal anatomical state, even though they were somewhat shrunken and mummified. Formalin gave off an odour which was unpleasant, pungent and distinctive. It went into our noses, got into our clothes and our eyes, and identified us as first-year students as it followed wherever we went during the first few weeks.

All of us had to purchase Cunningham's *Manual of Practical Anatomy*. This legendary three-volume text- copies of which I still have- was our Bible. It described every organ, vessel, nerve, muscle and bone in the body. In addition to this text, each batch had to have a set of dissection instruments. We were divided into ten-member groups and allotted a cadaver each. Our cadaver was male and naked. This was the first time any of us had seen a naked man. I opened my dissection kit and ran my fingers over the scalpel, forceps and scissors.

'Remove the skin flap of the lower limb, and expose the fascia, I'll come and explain the anatomy of it,' Professor Garg's voice boomed over us.

My group members and I looked at each other blankly. Not one of us knew how to even hold a scalpel, let alone using it for making an incision or exposing a skin flap. It was like a scene out of the popular Bollywood film, *Munna Bhai MBBS* and like the film, no one volunteered. Uncertainly, I stepped forward. I picked up the scalpel and tried to fix its blade. Professor Garg watched me struggle from a distance and then stepped in. He then verbally explained how to open a flap. 'You have 30 minutes,' he announced. I stepped closer to the cadaver, whose formalin smell made me nauseous. My eyes burned.

But shortly after, I found I had got used to it. I held the skin with forceps in my right hand, and with a scalpel in my left, I dissected the skin flap. Professor Garg was impressed. From then on, my peers pushed me forward every time there was a call for dissection. I would dissect 80 per cent of the cadaver. We did not wear gloves and the formalin wrinkled the skin on my fingers and hands. It taught me how it's the first step that is the toughest. What follows is not only easy, but can also be fun. Today, due to the paucity of bodies and limited spaces, anatomy is taught using computers, virtual reality and 3D printing. But in my view, dissecting a body from head to toe is the best way to learn anatomy.

Our physiology teachers, Dr B.B.L. Mathur (Dean), Dr S.S. Mishra Sr, Dr R.S. Pandey, Dr S.S. Mishra Jr, and Dr Kiran Patel were very good. But I found physiology practicals somewhat disagreeable. Almost invariably, we used a frog. We had to first 'pith' it—i.e. put a sharp, long instrument into its spinal cord to paralyze it below the neck. Even though it did not feel any pain thereafter, I found pithing inhumane and always got someone else to do it. I have to admit, though, that these practicals enabled us to thoroughly study the frog's muscle and cardiac activity, histology, which involved studying the microscopic structure of various tissues and organs and using different stains to make the tissues and organs stand out.

I wasn't nearly the best at everything. In histology class, the sight of multiple microscopes lined on a table terrified me. Stained tissue specimens were placed on slides and students were asked to focus the slides and appreciate the histology. My peers knew how to focus the microscope, I did not. I struggled with adjustment screws and slide positioning but as time would start to run out, I would have to ask for help. In no time, a tutor would arrive at my working station, showing me how the microscope worked. He also asked me to get my eyes checked, telling me that my eyesight should be perfect for me to effectively handle the microscope. Through these experiences, I not only learnt that there should be no hesitation in asking for help when it is needed, but also that when people see your enthusiasm to learn, they may go above and beyond to assist you. This is how it worked in my medical college and also in life—not everyone is able to learn all these lessons. But those who ask, show they are eager to learn and make a sincere effort, often receive the training few others do.

## The Tide Turns

As I left for my hostel after the histology class, I was happy and excited at the possibilities before me. Success until then had meant having plenty to eat at the end of the day, lying peacefully in my bed and anticipating the next day's lectures as mosquitoes buzzed around me while I tried to sleep. Most of the time, I cooked for myself and often skipped meals to save enough for college fees and hostel rent. When examinations were close, I would eat only one meal (a late lunch) at Jain Bhojanalaya (in front of the medical college) at 4 or 5 P.M. and this would serve as both my lunch and dinner. Our family was under great financial strain and this approach helped me save each and every penny I could out of what my father sent. Every day, I would wake up and write in my diary about the gift of 1,440 minutes given to me by God. I would decide to use this greatest gift of all, as wisely and efficiently as I could and resolved to use each and every rupee my parents sent to make them feel proud of me. And that would help me truly avenge them against all the misbehaviour. If I was able to achieve it, I would feel successful.

But as my professors showed faith in my abilities, my definition of success expanded. I became more ambitious, competitive, and goal-oriented. My biggest immediate goal was to stabilize my finances while doing well in my career. I wanted to prove myself before my relatives and childhood friends, who did not believe that I had any potential. As I got close to becoming a doctor, I drowned myself in studies further and strictly avoided all distractions. Unlike other students, partying was simply not an option for me. I had neither the money, nor the means. I stayed in the hostel and kept mostly to myself. I would only participate in group discussions when I wanted to understand abstruse topics and clear my doubts. I kept the company of seniors who generously helped me with my studies, lent me their books and treated me like their younger brother.

## Occupational Exposure: Tubercular Pleural Effusion

During my final year at MBBS, I started developing a low-grade fever every evening. I also noticed a mild cough and left-sided chest pain. When I consulted a physician, Dr B.N. Srivastava, he suggested a chest X-ray and a few blood tests to investigate the cause of the fever. To my surprise, the X-ray report revealed a left-sided pleural effusion! I was taken aback by the results as the most common cause of the pleural effusion is tuberculosis. Tubercular pleural effusion is the second most common form of extrapulmonary tuberculosis and a common cause of pleural effusions in endemic tuberculosis areas. I took anti-tubercular treatment (rifampicin, isoniazid, ethambutol) for one year. At the beginning of the treatment, I was also given the streptomycin injection for a few weeks. A follow-up X-ray revealed the thickened pleura, which was evidence of my body responding to treatment.

While working in hospitals, medical students, trainee doctors and medical professionals are exposed to several diseases including tuberculosis, HIV, Hepatitis B and C (as a result of sharp needle injury), and a variety of respiratory infections such as influenza and coronavirus. Later on, I came to know that my spouse and some of her colleagues at AIIMS, New Delhi had also been affected by tuberculosis. As medical professionals, we have a sense of the risks involved and yet we remain engaged, continuing to care for our patients. Perhaps society prefers to remain blissfully unaware of the sacrifice and risk doctors endure, taken in by the serenity of the hospital where the ill are nurtured back to health. Perhaps we are all loathe to let reality and data shatter this illusion.

In addition to contracting diseases, doctors also risk developing high stress from overworking, depression, hopelessness, burnout, restricted social life and are also prone to alcohol, drug abuse, drug exposure and suicide—this is not uncommon among medical students, resident doctors and medical professionals. The stress of balancing work and a social life remains a big challenge for many doctors. It is also common for patients' relatives to blame doctors for a poor prognosis of the disease. The constant threat of legal trouble and consumer cases add further to the stress of the job.

After talking to hundreds of medical students and young doctors, I realized that the worst part is that our systems are not equipped to prevent, treat or compensate or even acknowledge, sometimes, if these big issues plague the healers themselves. These occupational hazards are not known to aspiring doctors, nor are they discussed in medical colleges. Administrators and regulators refrain from collating and publishing data that would establish the risks involved in becoming a doctor or nurse. Some of these hazards may be known, but there is no comprehensive analysis of workplace risks for medical professionals, as there are for other professions. As medical professionals, we have a sense of the risk and yet we persevere, simply accepting that 'these things happen'.

Every day, globally, doctors and nurses return to their workplace to take care of their patients, knowing well the risks involved. It is time for us to acknowledge that doctors, nurses and healthcare workers run the constant risk of getting sick, injured, disabled or burdened with court cases as they care for their patients in the best manner. Doctors save the patient, but it is important for our society to also focus on the well-being of doctors.

## Studying in Hostel behind Locked Doors

I was accommodated at hostel number 1. My building was close to the medical college and provided us with excellent facilities. However, during the holidays, some colleagues or seniors would drop into my room to gossip about girls or teachers or have long discussions on religion or politics. This would disturb my study schedule and I wondered how I could avoid the intrusion. Dr Avadh Bihari Parashar was staying in TT room (Table Tennis room) number 1 and I was staying in the adjoining number 2. The window of the TT rooms was big and without any iron grille. To minimize visitors and study without any interruption, I would lock my room from the outside and enter the room through the big window. The visitor would see the lock hanging on my door and think that I am not available in the hostel and go away. I would do this on the weekends or during the holidays, and this would give me time to study and complete all my assignments without any interruptions and disturbances.

## Our Own 'Munna Bhai MBBS' and 'Circuit'

It was the end of 1990 and I was in the final year of my MBBS. Instead of going home for summer vacations, I decided to stay back and focus on my course. As a result, my medical knowledge and ability to diagnose ailments correctly, improved significantly. One day, my senior, Dr Devendra Pratap Singh (whom we called D.P. Singh sir) called me. He said, 'Pandey ji, I have received word from the hostel that you are doing well in your studies. If any medical student or teacher asks, tell them that D.P. Singh sir teaches you.'

D.P. Singh sir was definitely interested in teaching his junior medical students, but not necessarily in studying. When asked about any medical complication or rare disease, he would narrate the name, page number, line number of the medical book containing the right answer within a few seconds. We later found out, much to our amusement, that like in the films *Munna Bhai M.B.B.S.* and *Lage Raho Munna Bhai*, he had 'Circuits' feeding him all this information. In fact, most of the time, the questions were already predecided by his Circuits and the harmless aim behind it was to impress the new medical students, hoping to motivate them to memorize their textbooks as he appeared to have done. He constantly urged his students to empathize with the poor, feel their pain as their own and then provide them with healthcare. According to him, to become a successful doctor, it is necessary to have compassion in life and to experience the life of economically poor patients.

## Apple of the Eye

While studying at medical college, my entire focus was on studies and studies alone. Except for NCC camp, my participation in extracurricular activities, sports was almost nil. The environment at that time was such that the students doing other things apart from studies were considered irresponsible and careless by their family members. Now when I look back, I regret not being able to participate in extracurricular activities during my student life and consider it a deficiency when it comes to all-round personality development.

Extracurricular activities helped my classmates immensely. In fact, our faculty members, seniors and classmates appreciated students who knew how to sing, dance, participate in stage performances, anchoring, mimicry, etc. in the college. During the annual programme, such students would become the apples of everyone's eyes. One such person was my friend, Dr Anil Sureen. Dr Sureen practises medicine in Dubai and is world-renowned for his Neuro Linguistic Programming (NLP) courses. Dr Sureen told me that his involvement in extracurricular activities helped him become one of the most popular students in his class. Eventually, he also became friends with Dr Vinita Chaurasia, a classmate of ours, and the two eventually went on to tie the knot after a few years. He told me that the biggest diseases in life are hesitation and waiting for the perfect time to start important work. Doing this prevents people from doing what is important to them. Most people are very sensitive to criticism and they take people's negative comments very seriously. According to Dr Sureen, we should remember the song, *'kuch to log kehenge, logon ka kaam hai kehna'* ('people will always have something to say, that is their job'), and continue chasing our dreams.

## NCC Camp

In my second year, I had a chance to attend the NCC camp at Mandu (district Dhar) in June 1987. The opportunity improved my ability to work in a team and provided me with a lot of other learnings. I was one in a group of sixty enthusiastic medical students who stayed in a tent in a jungle near Mandu (Dhar, M.P.) for ten days. I learned how to dig a trench, fire safety measures, first aid, and also how to fire a gun. The routine for all of us was to get up early in the morning, have tea, parade and learn unity, punctuality, discipline and teamwork. I also learned the ABC of emergency management as well as giving first aid to trauma patients. After completing my training, I received a 'C' certificate in NCC. Professor H.K.T. Raza (an orthopaedic surgeon and former dean of Chhindwara Medical College) taught us a great deal during the camp. Professor Raza was one of the best teachers I had during my medical career and I remember him fondly. He was very fitness-conscious and instilled in us the great value of maintaining sound work ethics and extracurricular activities. Unfortunately, we lost our great teacher on 14 March 2019 to a massive myocardial infarction.*

---

* Jamal Ashraf, 'Prof. HKT Raza (1956–2019)', *Indian J Orthop*, May–June 2019, 53(3), p. 488. Available at: https://www.ncbi.nlm.nih.gov/pmc/articles/PMC6501633/.

# 4

# Academic Blitzkrieg

## Succeeding in Medical College

Despite all my efforts, a problem persisted. My marks remained low during the first-year MBBS examinations. After weeks of deliberating, I realized that the issue was very fundamental. It was the language of instruction. I had grown up being instructed in Hindi and now suddenly, I was in uncharted territory, surrounded by English. And I was drowning.

I was spending all my time researching, reading and making notes. But somehow, in the exam hall, I failed to find the right language to express myself. The more I tried, the more I lost control over words. It was as if I was slurring on paper. I decided to seek help and reached out to a college senior who, like me, had come from a Hindi-medium school. 'What do I do?' I asked him as we walked around the campus, passing by Indian Coffee House and taking in the hills visible at a distance.

'Have fun with the language,' he said. 'Use your imagination, use mnemonics'. He helped me memorize the names of the carpal bones

(Scaphoid, Lunate, Triquetrum, Pisiform and Trapezium, Trapezoid, Capitate and Hamate) using the simple mnemonic: '*Snehlata Tinde Paka, Tere Tinde Kachhe Hain.*' It was fairly simple advice but it unlocked something in me. Till then, I had been hard at work—beating myself up for every missed comma. Now I relaxed. I began to explore how to use keywords, associations, linkages and substitution techniques. I started playing around with mind maps, mnemonics and diagrams. This, combined with discussions with colleagues and seniors, helped me turn a new leaf. Within six months, I managed to emerge as one of the top 20 students in my class. Since my seniors had played such a key role in helping me get there, I was careful to teach and guide my juniors. Finally, all these extra efforts aided me in improving my rank to second in the class by my final year of MBBS.

## A Doctor in the Making

After passing the MBBS examination, the 12-month rotatory internship was mandatory before qualifying to practice independently as a doctor. We were paid a stipend of Rs 900 per month during the internship. In most of these postings, we filled forms and dressed wounds. Nothing was exciting. Patients also considered us trainees and did not take us seriously. However, I found the internship period to be very interesting. I could hang a stethoscope around my neck and learn from patients admitted to the hospital's medical or surgical wards, which I did with great enthusiasm.

A hospital can compel you to re-evaluate the meaning of the word 'emergency'. Every minute involved a race against time. Doctors would be on their feet for eighteen hours, without breaks or balanced meals. Sleep, savouring a cup of chai and leisurely reading the newspaper were but vague memories. The here and now was that patients were pouring in with a variety of ailments. NSCB Medical College Hospital was the biggest government hospital in Central India at the time and doctors and other healthcare staff scampered to find empty beds on a good day. On bad days, even chairs were in short supply. I, a 23-year-old intern, was in the middle of this chaos—the eye of the storm. I had been cruising through postings, from obstetrics and gynaecology to paediatrics, and currently, had now been posted in the emergency unit.

It was my third week. I had spent the first two weeks managing general emergencies and my seniors believed that I could now help with critical patients. My abilities were tested on 26 January 1991 when a patient was brought in critical condition. Despite the cold weather, he was sweating profusely. He was reeling under a myocardial infarction—a heart attack. Severe chest pain was shooting up to his left hand and the left side of his jaw. He was dizzy and could hardly breathe. I looked at him and gulped. I knew I had to act fast. But how? Looking at his case made me miss my days in the obstetrics and gynaecology department, where I had learnt how to deliver babies. I learnt how to cut the umbilical cord and hold and handle newborns, spent a lot of time going around blood banks as most patients were anaemic or lost a lot of blood and occasionally, I even had to convince sceptical family members and friends to donate blood and wipe their doubts.

But could I help a patient who was suffering from a heart attack? Could I ensure that a dying man was restored to life again? It was a moment of truth. I recalled the ABC of managing a medical emergency: Airway, Breathing and Circulation. I immediately put on the oxygen mask and started the oxygen. The next step was to record his vital parameters—pulse, blood pressure, oxygen saturation—and to immediately secure an intravenous line. I had seen nurses and emergency medical officers masterfully insert an intravenous cannula in a patient's vein to inject drugs. It was my turn to do it. I asked the ward attendant to hold the patient's hand tightly. I dabbed a spirit swab on the dorsum of the hand and tapped the vein. Without wasting any time, I carefully inserted the venflon in the vein and covered it with the cannula fixing tape. I quickly injected the intravenous fluid with medicines to control pain. I also asked him to put a nitroglycerine tablet under his tongue to increase the blood supply in the vessels supplying the heart, and meanwhile, an electrocardiogram (ECG) technician and cardiologist were urgently called. I took a few steps back as they arrived and took charge of the case. The patient was now more comfortable.

His family was elated. They all thanked me profusely, brought me sweets, and promised to visit me in my private clinic whenever I had one. I was ecstatic but told them I was merely a junior doctor. I had always been shy. I never thought I would enjoy interacting with patients or their kin. But the internship changed everything. There were days when even eighteen hours of duty didn't tire me. In fact, I couldn't wait to reach the hospital and start work on most days. Those eighteen hours were often blissful, a time when I could set my personal problems aside. Many medical students shy away from completing their internships or are too busy preparing for the NEET PG examination. But in doing so, they miss out on the experience of functioning as a doctor. My internship taught me that you can be a medical graduate by force, but never a doctor. You can become a doctor only by choice. See yourself as the only one between a patient's life and their grave, and you'll find all the motivation you need to start taking initiative from day one.

## Secret Rounds in the Hospital Ward

However, the internship wasn't all I was doing at the time. I was also nurturing dreams of pursuing a postgraduate degree in ophthalmology. I had started training for it long ago. As an MBBS student, I would often accompany my senior, Dr M. Yusuf Rizvi (now working as the head of the department, ophthalmology, Government Doon Medical College, Dehradun, Uttarakhand), for his evening rounds in the eye wards. He was completing his Master's of Surgery in Ophthalmology at the time. Dr Rizvi encouraged my curiosity and patiently explained the clinical details of a variety of cases to me. I did not know back then but Dr Rizvi's teachings were preparing me for a career in ophthalmology long before I took up the formal education.

During one of our clinical postings, twenty classmates and I wore white aprons, nameplates, hung stethoscopes around our necks and followed our professor, Dr Vijay Bhaisare, to the OPD. It was Dr Bhaisare's first posting after his training at Dr R.P. Centre for Ophthalmic Sciences, AIIMS, New Delhi. Many eye patients had been admitted to the ward and Dr Bhaisare was examining an interesting case of severe dry eyes caused due to an allergy to sulfa drugs. He asked us for our diagnoses. My classmates were unsure. Many said they didn't know. I was standing behind, closely observing the patient. 'Steven Johnson Syndrome,' I said. Dr Bhaisare asked me to come forward and explain what I was talking about. I told him that this was a type of drug-induced allergic reaction that caused the skin to blister and peel off. My classmates were surprised. They looked at me curiously, as if asking how I had been able to diagnose a syndrome they had never even heard of. They didn't know about my secret rounds with Dr Rizvi.

When my internship had begun, I had decided to start preparing for the Pre-PG examination. I believed I had an edge as I had been residing with seniors who were pursuing postgraduate degrees in surgery, paediatrics and medicine, among other fields. I could easily approach them for clinical or other queries. I found that the best way to clarify my doubts was to accompany my seniors on their ward rounds during the evenings, where they could show me and explain clinical cases to me hands-on. But this was hardly the end of my preparation. Every night after dinner, after all those hours of gruelling work at the hospital, I would sit with other students to prepare for exams. We would shoot rapid-fire questions at each other to help us retain the information. On weekends, we would practise through mock tests. These efforts paid off, as when the results came, I ranked seventh in the state pre-PG examination.

Despite my academic success and now a confirmed seat in ophthalmology at NSCB Medical College, Jabalpur, a nagging feeling gripped me. The achievement, I realized, was not nearly enough. I wanted to pursue PG where I would have access to modern tools and technology. This place wasn't it. Almost all cases were examined under the light of a flashlight in the Eye OPD. The slit lamp, which should have been used, was kept in the room of Professor Ashok K. Mukherjee (chief of the eye department), who did not want to risk accidental damage and hence, did not allow resident doctors to use it. This led to a lot of difficulties in making accurate diagnoses; such as between acute conjunctivitis and acute uveitis.

One day, I asked a senior, Dr Dinesh Sahu, who had returned to Jabalpur after pursuing a fellowship from Aravind Eye Hospital, Madurai, how to make that distinction using a flashlight. He taught me how to look for 'cells' in the anterior chamber and for the first time ever, I saw hundreds of tiny cells shining like stars on a dark night. I knew I would've been reprimanded for trying to go too far too soon instead of focusing on completing my MS first. But I wasn't ready to wait. It was clear to me that you needed to use the right equipment to explore the pathology and appreciate the beauty of a 2.5 cm organ. I realized then that for the learning I sought, I needed to pursue my specialization from a more renowned medical institution like the Post Graduate Institute of Medical Education and Research (PGIMER), Chandigarh, or the All India Institute of Medical Sciences (AIIMS), New Delhi. But I had already secured admission at NSCB Medical College. I was at a crossroads, and I didn't know what to do. Was it worth trying for a residency all over again? What if I did not get a seat in a premier college and wasted precious time in the ongoing residency as well? Pursuing a residency and preparing for Pre-PG is like sailing in two boats at once and I simply didn't know if I had it in me to do it.

## Flash of Light

A few months had passed since I started my PG. It was the month of November and Diwali was around the corner. But I didn't want to go home, so I decided to stay on at my institute and spend time in the library instead. On the day of Diwali, while reading an old issue of the *Indian Journal of Ophthalmology*, I came across a very interesting article. It was about Dr Sohan Singh Hayreh.[*]

Dr Hayreh came from a family under high financial stress. His father, along with several other servicemen from the state of Patiala, was given compulsory early retirement. His pension was inadequate to support the family of five children. I was hooked. Dr Hayreh's background was just like mine. He came from a village where everyday life was riddled with struggle. Like me, he wanted to pursue a career in academic research, but had little to no access to suitable opportunities. He finally decided to complete his medical degree and join the Indian Army, where the pay was decent. But he loathed the regimentation and subordination. Every day, he waited to complete his army contract and eventually rose through the ranks in academia to join a prestigious university in the US.

I was so affected by his story and our similarities that I could not sleep that night. The more I thought about it, the more I realized that it was no coincidence that I was reading this on the day of Diwali. His story enlightened me and showed me a path. I had to strive for brilliance. I promised myself that I would try harder to achieve my dreams, even if that meant dropping out of my current course and trying for another one. I placed the photo of Dr Sohan Singh Hayreh in my room and began to consider him my guru.[†]

---

[*] S.S. Hayreh, 'Remembrances of things past', Indian Journal of Ophthalmology, 39, pp. 140–6, 1991. Available at: https://www.ijo.in/text.asp?1991/39/3/140/24447.

[†] I was lucky to meet and interact with Dr Hayreh three times during my stay in the USA. He was very happy to learn that his biography solved my dilemma and motivated me to become a successful eye surgeon.

I felt ready to work with renewed energy. I started to juice each minute of each day. I began to carry my books to the ophthalmology ward. Late-night rapid fires and mock exams on the weekends began again. I examined patients and studied. There was no time for anything else. Yet, one day, I had to make time for a worrisome meeting.

Someone from the department had conveyed my intention of preparing for the entrance examination for pursuing my PG at premier eye institutions (AIIMS, New Delhi, PGIMER, Chandigarh) to Professor Mukherjee. He summoned me. I walked into his large office that most residents religiously avoided. He crossed his arms over his large glass-top table and glared at me. 'Why do you want to waste your seat?' he yelled. He commanded me to focus on my work or face grave consequences.

My heart sank. It was a clear warning and I thought that was that and I would have to give up my desire to study at PGIMER, Chandigarh. My parents also suggested that I stay in Jabalpur. I spent many days mulling over it, drawing chits and picking fingers. But then I thought back to my childhood, to the day when I had recited Dr A.P.J. Abdul Kalam before everyone in class. And then I thought about my new ideas of success, and the decision was clear. The pieces were beginning to fall into place.

# 5

# Lightning Bolt

## Learning to Punch Above My Weight

*'If you believe in yourself and have dedication and pride and never quit, you'll
be a winner. The price of victory is high but so are the rewards.'*

—Paul Bryant

Towards the end of 1994, I left Jabalpur for Chandigarh, a city
planned by the French architect Le Corbusier. However, it is said
to be an extension of an earlier design by an American architect,
Albert Mayor. I hopped onto an overnight bus at the Interstate
Bus Terminus (ISBT), Delhi. It was a dark, lonesome night and
I was blissfully unaware of the terror that lay in waiting along
the way. When I arrived, I was admonished for taking the bus
by Superintendent of Police (SP) Ajay Pandey, (who was working
together with DGP Punjab Late K.P.S. Gill to crush militancy),
a family friend, asked me, 'Don't you know that terrorists are
more likely to target non-Sikh travellers on the road?' I didn't but
perhaps even that knowledge wouldn't have stopped me from
joining the three-year residency programme for Master of Surgery
in Ophthalmology at the prestigious PGIMER, Chandigarh. The

institute was established in 1962 and situated in Sector 12 in front of Punjab University situated in Sector 14.* Its three founders, Dr Tulsi Das, Dr Santokh Singh Anand, and Dr P.N. Chhuttani, were all from Amritsar Medical College and approached the Government of India to set up the PGIMER. Sardar Partap Singh Kairon, the then Chief Minister of Punjab, went to PM Jawaharlal Nehru about the matter and he agreed.

## '*Tobe Ekla Chalo Re*'

I hailed an auto from the bus stand and was struck by how spacious and clean Chandigarh was. Throughout my journey, Rabindranath Tagore's words '*Tobe Ekla Chalo Re*' ('Do what is right even if you are alone on your path') rang in my ears. Despite my best efforts, my parents had failed to understand why I was quitting my residency in NSCB Jabalpur to go to Chandigarh. They were not alone. Anyone would have admonished me for dropping out of one well-respected course for another. But I had my eyes set on a goal far bigger than the government jobs or incremental achievements I was headed towards. The auto brought me to the PGIMER campus. As soon as we entered through the main gate, I asked my auto driver to stop for a few seconds. Engraved in golden letters were the Sanskrit words: 'आर्त सेवा सर्वभद्रः शोधश च' ('Service to the community, care of the needy and research for the good of all'). I beamed with pride.

I moved into room number C12, Old Doctors' Hostel (ODH), which was surrounded by lush green trees. I was happy to meet three doctors, Dr Rakesh Jindal, Dr Dheeraj Kamra, Dr Nishith Bhardwaj, from my own state of Rajasthan. There, as I got to know my ophthalmology colleagues, I realized that I had an advantage over them: the few months of experience in ophthalmology in Jabalpur.

---

* *The sectors in Chandigarh don't have the number 13! Since it was planned by a French architect, the inauspicious 13 was never part of the city.*

From the very first day, I would arrive at the hospital fully armed with a flashlight, a direct ophthalmoscope to observe the retina of the eye, and a 90 dioptre lens to examine the retina on a slit lamp. Among my first assignments was assisting Professor Jagjit S. Saini in completing a corneal transplantation.

After the cornea transplant surgery, Dr Saini was taking a ward round during the late evening hours. Senior residents, junior residents and a few junior faculty members accompanied him on his rounds. Dr Yadavinder P. Dang, a visiting faculty from the USA and PGI alumnus, also joined rounds to teach residents. Suddenly, the sister-in-charge of the ward requested him to examine a patient's attendant, who had developed diplopia or double vision. Professor Saini quickly flashed light in his eyes and noticed the drooping of both eyelids (also known as ptosis). The patient confirmed that as the day progressed, his eyelids drooped. Professor Saini used this as an opportunity to train his students and juniors. He asked us for a spot diagnosis.

'Myasthenia gravis,' I said.

'How can it be confirmed?' he asked.

'By the Tensilon Test,' my colleague answered. 'The test involves administering an injection of Tensilon (edrophonium), after which muscle strength is evaluated to determine whether the weakness is caused by myasthenia gravis or not.'

But Professor Saini was in a fun mood. 'Which famous film star had the same problem?' he asked.

This time, most of us knew the answer. 'Amitabh Bachchan,' we said.

My time at PGIMER, Chandigarh was exceptionally stimulating. Every day, I would see a variety of cases. Patients would come not only from Punjab and Haryana but also from neighbouring states such as Uttarakhand, Himachal Pradesh, Uttar Pradesh, Rajasthan, Jammu and Kashmir, etc. Some of them come with marked diminution or loss of vision and a retinal examination would reveal diabetic retinopathy or Grade III or Grade IV of hypertension-related changes in the retina. These changes sometimes suggested that the patient had uncontrolled diabetes or high blood pressure, but most patients would be unaware of having those conditions at all.

All these findings strengthened my belief that the eyes were not only the window to the soul—but to the body. Eye doctors can tell a lot about the overall health of the individual just by looking at their eyes. That's because the eye is the only place in the body that provides an unobstructed view of blood vessels, nerves and connecting tissue. As a result, eye examinations and tests can provide earlier diagnoses of diabetes, high blood pressure, cancer, multiple sclerosis, and many other conditions.

It was at PGIMER, Chandigarh that I learnt that perhaps doctors don't have all the solutions. One day, while I was on emergency duty, a fifty-three-year-old patient came with a complaint of sudden loss of vision. I examined them with an instrument called ophthalmoscope and saw central retinal artery occlusion (CRAO) or the blockage of the artery that supplies blood to the retina. To clear the passage of the tiny blood vessel, I immediately performed paracentesis, which required me to drain aqueous fluid using a 26 Gauge needle. Unfortunately, the patient did not gain their vision despite my best efforts. I was upset for many days over this but I had to keep reminding myself that I had done my best.

## The All India Ophthalmology Society Conference

My MBBS friends, resident colleagues and I would often talk about our work. Sometimes, my medicine or surgery resident colleagues would be surprised to see me in the ward for a fundus examination at odd hours. Most of them were under the impression that there is less clinical load and not many emergencies in ophthalmology. Most of our conversations would end with the same harmless joke. They would tease me for my work and remark at how I had dedicated my entire life to a 2.5 cm organ. 'You have no idea what you're talking about,' I once told them. 'Eyes are the windows to the body.' My friends didn't know that there was glamour attached to my job too, and the All India Ophthalmology Society (AIOS) Conference (February 3-6, 1996) at PGIMER showed them as much.

The conference was not just about boring speeches and panel discussions—doctors would perform live surgeries in front of an audience. Renowned eye surgeons from all over the world had come to Chandigarh on the occasion to perform live cataract (phacoemulsification) surgery and intraocular lens implantation, including Dr Keiki R. Mehta, Dr Abhay R. Vasavada, Dr Kumar J. Doctor, Dr N.V. Arulmozhi Varman and Dr Mahipal S. Sachdev. I was asked to get the cataract patients ready. I helped with the arrangements, then rushed to the operation theatre. I watched the live surgeries relayed from the operation theatre to Bhargava Auditorium in the PGIMER campus with unhidden fascination. There was only one thought in my head—when would I get to perform a live surgery? The opportunity would come nine years later at the International Ophthalmology Conference in Milan, Italy.

The All India Ophthalmological Society conference, a highly successful four-day mega event, was a proud moment for our chairman and chief organizing secretary Professor Amod Gupta, all faculty members, and residents of PGIMER, Chandigarh. A few eye doctors from Pakistan participating in this conference learned the art of phacoemulsification surgery in the Wet Lab that was held for the first time in the history of AIOS under the leadership of Professor Jagat Ram. Prominent national media published news quoting Indian eye doctors had already mastered the art of stitchless cataract surgery while Pakistani doctors were learning from them in the Wet Lab during the AIOS conference held at Chandigarh.

## Missing Lunch, Mentors and Training at PGIMER

For the most part, however, my time at PGIMER, Chandigarh, was spent treating patients, reading and learning. I would start my ward rounds at 7.00 A.M. Then from 9 A.M. to 5 P.M., I would work in the OPD and OT. I would participate in academic activities, discussions with faculty members and seniors from 5–7 P.M. Then once again, take a ward round from 7–9 P.M. to complete all the patient work. Then finally, after dinner at 9.30 P.M., I would go to the Dr Tulsi Das library to read the latest medical/ophthalmology journals or prepare for academic activities such as case presentations, journal clubs, staff clinical meetings, among others. The library was named after Dr Tulsi Das, a world-renowned ophthalmologist, the first director of PGIMER, Chandigarh and one of the founders of the institute. Most doctors didn't pause for lunch and at first, I found it challenging to comply.

One afternoon, my senior resident Dr Mrinal Anand, called for me to examine a multi-trauma emergency case. After examining the eyes of the patient and filing my notes, I rushed to a cafe for a quick lunch. I missed the food in Jabalpur, especially the Sunday feast of puri, kheer and halwa, but I found a place that served basic food. When I was returning, Dr Anand stopped me. 'You could have informed me,' he said. 'It's basic courtesy'. I was taken aback. Since that day, I made it a point to eat a heavy breakfast, carry biscuits for my rumbling stomach, but not leave the hospital for lunch no matter how famished I was.

To add to my travails, I couldn't speak Punjabi. When a patient visited me for a vision exam and asked to read the letters in Gurmukhi, I turned the chart but sat there clueless about what he was reading. Slowly, with the help of colleagues, and many scribbled notes and pocket dictionaries, I learnt Punjabi. I once asked Professor Mangat R. Dogra, the vitreo-retinal surgeon, whom I had always seen work in the Retinopathy of Prematurity (ROP) clinic without a break from

9 A.M. to 5 P.M., how he did it. 'I enjoy my work,' he smiled. 'I love working with infants. Besides, the parents of these babies come from faraway places—Himachal Pradesh, Jammu and Kashmir, Uttar Pradesh, Uttarakhand, Haryana—just to see me. I want to help them so they can live without going blind.' It was a simple but profound lesson. Professor Dogra enjoyed his work but along with that, he felt a sense of responsibility towards his patients which kept pushing him to do more.

I learned the art and science of ophthalmology from my excellent mentors at PGIMER, Chandigarh. These included Dr Amod Gupta (chairman), Late Dr Jagjit S. Saini, Dr Jagat Ram, Dr Mangat R. Dogra, Dr Kanwar Mohan, Dr Arun Kumar Jain, Dr Ashok Sharma, Dr S.S. Pandav, Dr Usha Singh. Professor Jagat Ram, past director, PGIMER, Chandigarh, was very popular among both the patients, as well as the residents. He was also my thesis guide. I considered him my ideal role model, who inspired me the most. His simplicity, compassionate behaviour with patients, his way of listening to the patients' complaints without interrupting them, his ability to stay calm during stressful situations and encouraging each and every resident to bring out the best in everyone in the team made for important lessons. It was doctors like them who inspired me to do more. So after my duty at the hospital, I would participate in grand rounds where I would present the medical problems and treatment of a particular patient to faculty members, senior residents and junior residents. I was also a regular at the journal club where we would critically evaluate recent articles in scientific journals.

I was deeply enriched by the academic environment at PGIMER, Chandigarh, where chairperson Dr Amod Gupta and faculty members would ask pointed questions related to clinical examination, differential diagnosis and emphasize bedside etiquette in ophthalmology. They did not blindly follow the recommendations of the western world without examining their relevance to our population, data or past experiences. The emphasis on publications and presentations during national and international conferences not only helped me grasp my subject better but also gave me enormous confidence to deliver scientific lectures.

## Under the Spotlight

Many renowned ophthalmologists visited PGIMER, Chandigarh at regular intervals. These included Dr Vinod Lakhanpal, Dr Verinder S. Nirankari, Dr Nursing A. Rao, Dr Suresh Chandra, Dr Emmett T. Cunningham, Dr Lingam Gopal, Dr Ken K. Nischal, Dr Jaswant S. Pannu, Dr Anita Agarwal, Dr Gullapalli Nageswara Rao, Dr Yadavinder P. Dang, Dr Sumit Nanda, etc. I recall one of the guest lectures that was delivered by Dr Sumit Nanda from the USA. Dr Nanda told Professor Amod Gupta, who was coordinating with him, that he would be presenting some unusual retinal cases that would be completely new for residents in India. Professor Gupta took this as a challenge and asked us residents to collect (and present) a series of unusual retina cases.

My case was a six-year-old girl who was suffering from eye cancer called retinoblastoma but was treated by a doctor who thought it was a case of uveitis or an inflammation of the eye. Sometimes this deadly cancer can masquerade as an inflammatory disease. And, that is what had happened in this case. This case had been referred to the eye department of PGIMER, Chandigarh by an eye surgeon in Jammu and Kashmir. The child had a remarkable decrease in vision in her right eye. When I investigated, I found that the right eye would have to be removed. But, it turned out to be impossible to convince her parents. After a week of strenuous efforts, of explaining to her parents that we feared the cancer would spread to the brain and lungs, they agreed.

When I presented my case, I was heartily appreciated by my colleagues and seniors because of how common the misdiagnosis is.

In a 1969 study by Stafford et al.,* nearly 40 per cent of patients with retinoblastoma had been initially misdiagnosed as having uveitis. Correct diagnosis can significantly avoid the mortality associated with this cancer. Just like in the case of this six-year-old girl.

This led to immediate gratification, which propelled me to keep working. As James Clear writes in his book, *Atomic Habits*, the brain needs an incentive to keep pursuing something—what better incentive than gratification? It was experiences like these that made the three years of my residency the most glorious years of my life. The emphasis on meticulous clinical examination, documentation and research-oriented teaching sent a clear message that I follow to date: observe, document, publish.

## The Eyes are Listening: A Squint Surgeon's Love for Santoor

In PGIMER, Chandigarh, I had the chance to learn the art and science of strabismus from Dr Kanwar Mohan. He was a respected faculty member at the Squint Unit, Ophthalmology department, PGIMER, Chandigarh, and trained by Professor Inder Sen Jain and other faculty members. Dr Mohan was very musically inclined and a disciple of the world-famous Santoor player, Pandit Shivkumar Sharma. Dr Mohan, too, played the santoor and always made it a point to attend his guru's performances during his visit to Chandigarh.

I greatly admired Dr Mohan's dedication and knowledge of the complex subject of squint and the perfection of his strabismus surgery technique. I asked him how he decided to dedicate his entire career to strabismus and he told me, 'when Professor Amod Gupta was allocating a subspecialty in ophthalmology, no faculty member was interested in taking up strabismus. So I decided to opt

---

* W.R. Stafford, M. Yanoff, B.L. Parnell, 'Retinoblastomas initially misdiagnosed as primary ocular inflammations', *Archives of Ophthalmology*, 82(6), 1969, pp. 771–773.

for strabismus and told Professor Gupta that I would dedicate my entire life to squint.'

In addition to squint surgery, I also learnt about meticulous record-keeping by taking preoperative and postoperative photos of strabismus patients. Most importantly, perhaps, my interaction with Dr Mohan taught me that practice makes perfect.

## A Fax for Matrimony

I was initially staying at Old Doctors' Hostel and later on, shifted to the Kairon block on the fifth floor of the PGIMER campus. The block was named after Late Sardar Partap Singh Kairon, then Chief Minister of Punjab; the other blocks were also named after the distinguished medical educationists of the then combined state of Punjab. PGIMER, Chandigarh owes its inception to the former CM's vision.

My elder sister had floated my matrimonial advertisement and had supplied my hostel address for responses—of which there were many. I had to fix up a wooden box in front of my room to receive these letters. One day, I got a twenty-page fax from the US. This fax contained the biodata of the girl and her parents. The PA to our HOD, Professor Amod Gupta, Jagjeet Singh Saini, called me to his office. He laughed and asked me, 'What's this? See, the paper is finished and we cannot receive any important fax now!' He then told me not to give out the department fax number in the future. When I visited Chandigarh in November 2021, to bid farewell to Professor Jagat Ram (former Director, PGIMER), a few of my friends recalled the letter box incident and we had a hearty laugh, as did Mr Saini.

# 6

# Unleashing My Potential

## On the Way to Becoming a Well-Rounded Doctor

*'Self-discipline is an act of cultivation. It requires you to connect today's actions to tomorrow's results. There's a season for sowing, a season for reaping. Self-discipline helps you know which is which.'*

—Gary Ryan Blair

## My First Research Project

In May 1996, Haryana Chief Minister Bhajan Lal sent a child from his family to the Eye OPD of PGIMER, Chandigarh. The twelve-year-old was suffering from a severe ocular allergy known as vernal kerato-conjunctivitis (VKC). The allergy was known to worsen in hot weather and dusty environments which would cause the child to rub his eyes vigorously. This, in turn, would deteriorate the condition further. Vigorous rubbing could threaten the development of a non-healing corneal ulcer (known as shield ulcer) as well as the weakening of the cornea, leading to protrusion or bulging of the cornea (known as keratoconus). The child had severe vision problems, including blurring of vision, double vision, ghost images, etc. When I saw this case, I was at a loss because there was no significant treatment for giant papillae and severe VKC cases available at the time. Eye drops would be helpful for transient relief. The market was flushed with steroid eye drops. Unsupervised self-administration of eye drops would often lead to cataract and/or glaucoma. Some of these children would develop giant papillae known as 'cobblestone follicles' inside the upper eyelids, causing intense itching, foreign body sensation, ropy discharge, and poor vision.

I mulled over the child's case for days, rummaging for case histories in the library. One day, I came across the latest March 1996 issue of the *American Journal of Ophthalmology*. A new paper from the Proctor Foundation for Research in Ophthalmology, University of California, discussed how supratarsal injection of steroids managed resistant or recalcitrant cases of VKC.*

I was unable to sleep that night. I took a photocopy of the article and marched to the office of the in-charge of the cornea unit, Professor Jagjit Singh Saini, first thing in the morning. I wrote a research plan to compare the efficacy of supratarsal injection. But I wanted to take it a notch further, so I focused on the short-acting dexamethasone sodium phosphate versus the intermediate-acting triamcinolone acetonide. Professor Saini gave us the go-ahead and we administered the child with the injection. Within three to four days after the supratarsal injection, the cobblestone papilla regressed, the shield ulcer disappeared gradually and the child's desire to itch subsided. Parallelly, we also continued our research, which had remarkable results. We completed a one-year follow-up and the outcome of our research on forty eyes was published in the *Acta Ophthalmological International Journal of Ophthalmology* in its January 1999 issue.

---

* D.S. Holsclaw DS, et al, 'Supratarsal injection of corticosteroid in the treatment of refractory vernal keratoconjunctivitis', American Journal of Ophthalmology, March 1996, 121(3), pp. 243–9. doi: 10.1016/s0002-9394(14)70271-5. PMID: 8597266.

## Failure at Close Quarters

Not all research experiences were as remarkable. In the first year, I spent a lot of time writing a case report on tuberculosis of the lacrimal gland. I did extensive reading and research in the library, wrote and rewrote the manuscript several times and sent it to the *Journal of Paediatric Ophthalmology and Strabismus* for publication.*

After a few weeks, word was sent that a fax had arrived for me. I rushed to the office and saw a rejection email from the publication. Rejections sting, but this one was particularly brutal. They wrote that not only did my work not add anything new to the existing literature, but the draft was filled with grammatical errors. I was crestfallen. My mentor, Dr Ashok Sharma, consoled me and told me that rejections were routine. Most papers, he said, get rejected a few times before they are finally published. But he did advise me to seek help to improve my English by getting the manuscript carefully read by another colleague or by a professional editor. I agreed with him and decided to act on my weakness.

A few hours passed when another fax arrived in my name. How odd of them, I thought, to send two faxes to convey news of the same rejection. It felt like rubbing salt on my wounds. I was in no hurry to collect the rejection fax once again, so I took my time to finish my work before I got to it. When I eventually reached the office and read the fax, I had to read it again and again. Within a span of a few hours, the editorial office had changed their decision. They had now faxed to inform us that they would publish the paper since it was the first report on tuberculosis of the lacrimal gland in a ten-year-old child and that they would correct the English at their end. I couldn't believe what I was reading. I also learnt a very important lesson—if your work is good, language is not a barrier to success.

---

* A. Sharma, S.K. Pandey, et al, 'Tuberculosis of the lacrimal gland: a case report', *Journal of Pediatric Ophthalmology Strabismus*, July–August 1998, 35(4), pp. 237–9. doi: 10.3928/0191-3913-19980701-14. PMID: 9713800.

Many researchers in India face problems in their careers because of their poor English. In addition to the language barrier, I also had the habit of speaking too fast. While I would urge everyone to learn English as well as they could and become fluent in the language, they must remember that language can be fixed, but poor work and ethics cannot.

To improve my English, I found it helpful to read a lot—from magazines to newspapers. I developed a habit of reading books and scientific journals regularly and enjoy learning new words. I started speaking in English during my morning motivational video sessions while cycling. This helped me to speak slowly, clearly, and with confidence on various topics other than ophthalmology.

## No Two Days are the Same

While research and surgery were an important part of my job, activities that I naturally gravitated towards, being a doctor involves much more. As a first-year resident, my job was to hand over the sample that was collected from several cases of eye infection to the microbiology department. This meant running from one building to the third or fifth floor of another. After two days or so, I was to collect the report and give it to the senior resident. Many newly joined residents were unhappy with this and they would call it 'donkey work' or 'scut work'.* I wasn't a big fan of running between buildings either, but slowly, I got used to it. I realized that this work gave me an opportunity to maintain touch with microbiologists and learn more about their work. Eventually, we even authored a few research publications together.

But running around, coupled with long hours of working definitely impacted my health. I was underweight, barely 48 kgs

---

* While the definition of scut work varies among individual residents, it generally refers to any task that can be completed by an employee without a medical degree.

for my 5 feet 8 inch stature. A nurse once looked at me and said, 'Dr Pandey, you should eat well or you will look like you're starving yourself.' I thought she was absolutely correct. If I didn't look like I took care of my own health, why would patients come to me? To top it all, I was in Punjab, where the patients were tall and well-built. I decided to do something about my weight. However, the rigorous hours at the hospital foiled all my efforts.

A rather strange idea came to mind. I rushed to the washroom and looked at myself in the mirror. It was winter so I was wearing a sweater over my shirt. 'Why not reverse this?' I thought. Let's wear a sweater or maybe two sweaters and then a shirt. Then I looked at my legs. Maybe I can wear a pair of jeans and then my loose trousers. I thought this was a brilliant plan. Clothes could mask my physique till I actually put on weight. I brought the method into effect the next day. But it was a half-baked plan. I had not thought it through. One day, I was putting on civil clothes in the changing room after finishing surgery when a colleague walked in. 'Why are you wearing another pair of trousers over those jeans?' he asked. I was caught red-handed. I couldn't think of any excuse so I told him the truth. Within a few hours, I had become a laughing stock in the hospital and for days to come, everyone who met me, asked, 'So, Dr Pandey, how many trousers are you wearing today?'

## Early Lesson for Becoming a Successful Doctor

Sometimes, working with patients is less about medicine and more about behaviour management. I was glad that word of my antics didn't reach my patients who, if unbothered by a starving doctor, would definitely have been bothered by the idea of being treated by a double-trousered doctor. Besides, I had worked hard to build a good rapport with my patients, who often had to wait long hours for a consultation. Sometimes, up to 400 patients would arrive at the hospital and each patient would have to wait an inordinate amount of time to meet with a doctor.

One day, a patient lost his temper due to the prolonged waiting. He tore up his OPD card. I lost my temper, too. I pointed him to the dustbin and asked him to throw the bits in it and follow the exit sign and leave the OPD. This kind of argument was common among junior residents, but senior doctors were far more patient. One day, Dr Rajan Shonek noticed a similar incident. Once again, I had lost my temper. He called me aside and asked me what the matter was. I told him that a few patients would get aggressive and start fighting. I, too, would sometimes get impatient. Dr Shonek sighed, took me to the side and said, 'They may lose their temper, but you shouldn't'. Dr Shonek suggested that I never take the patients' complaints personally.

'This is a part of the life of a healer, Suresh,' he said. 'Why are you annoyed? You should be happy that you are surrounded by so many patients. You should learn to listen to the patient without interrupting them, and try to solve their problem as soon as possible.' I had never thought that my existence depended on my patients and that I was getting impatient with those who I was meant to help. This conversation taught me a very important lesson for life. I made a promise to myself that I would try my best to control my temper, even if the patient provokes me or is unreasonable. Dr Shonek's lesson has stayed with me, and we've remained great friends.* I now realize that this was the most important that which helped me become a successful and popular doctor. Many doctors with the most seasoned surgical skills and outstanding clinical acumen never explore their complete potential as successful or famous doctors due to one limitation—they are short-tempered, easily provoked and unable to listen to their patients without interruptions. I was glad to have learnt this lesson early in life.

---

* Dr Rajan Shonek is currently practising in Patiala and visited me in Kota in 2017 to learn the secret of high-volume ophthalmic practice.

Today, after having treated more than 15 lakh patients and completing more than 1 lakh eye surgeries, the most important lesson that I have learned is that you may encounter happy, unhappy and angry patients. You need to be a good listener and never lose your calm. Devote time to addressing the problem. Time is the best healer. Most patients accept the new diagnoses or complications after a gap of a few weeks or a few months.

Get sound sleep, exercise and meditate regularly, and eat healthy. These things also give you a feeling of control and minimize anger. Anger is a normal and healthy emotion, but being short-tempered and spiralling out of control over small things does not only negatively impact you but also the people around you. So you have to learn to control your anger. I found it helpful to follow these rules:

- If you feel your temper rising, move away from that place. Take a deep breath or go for a walk. It can calm you down.
- When you become angry, try imagining a place where you feel happy and calm.
- Try a new hobby like dancing, running, singing etc. to distract yourself from your annoyance. This is a great way to let go of your anger and feel relaxed.
- Exercise every day or practice meditation, which can help you channel your anger more effectively.
- Count from one to ten before you respond to an angry or unreasonable patient.
- Smile when you feel your temper rising—this goes a long way in cooling down the situation.
- Surround yourself with calming scents to soothe your nerves.
- Write down everything when you feel angry and re-read it once a week. Once you start writing down your feelings of anger, you will observe your temper automatically subsiding.

## Knocked Down

By December 1997, I was close to finishing my junior residency. I believed I was in a good place. I was considered to be a sincere and hardworking resident who had five national and two international publications in peer-reviewed journals, and four paper presentations to his credit. I was perhaps among the few junior residents to achieve such a feat. I decided to apply for senior residency at the same institute. A senior residency or fellowship is crucial in surgical branches as it provides experience and surgical exposure, and imparts you the skills required to move out of an institute and start practising independently. I was confident that I would make it. I wanted to gain more surgical experience in the field of ophthalmology, particularly anterior segment ophthalmology. I was confident that the exemplary staff at PGIMER, Chandigarh would help me master the art of eye surgery.

However, only two positions were available. When the results were announced, I was heartbroken—I had not been given the position. The news not only disappointed me but also came as a shock to my mentor, Professor Jagat Ram. 'Be patient,' he told me, 'and keep working with enthusiasm. When God closes a door, He opens a window of opportunity. There may be something better waiting for you.'

I had lost my chance to work at PGIMER, Chandigarh, but I had to keep trying. I started applying to other institutes and was selected for the position of a senior resident at the Department of Ophthalmology, Government Medical College, Chandigarh. But it wasn't my dream institute. Something was missing. I had spent hours reading through the work of Indian ophthalmologists who had excelled in their fields. I read about the unusual journey of some of the ophthalmologists of Indian origin who did remarkable work and became world-renowned researchers. These included Dr Sohan Singh Hayreh, Dr Prashant Kumar Basu, Dr Narsing A. Rao, Dr

Harminder S. Dua, etc. During this time (in 1998), I had written a letter to Dr Narsing A. Rao asking him about the secrets of becoming a successful researcher at Doheny Eye Institute, UCLA Stein Eye Institute, Los Angeles, California, USA and was very happy to receive his encouraging reply and pearls of wisdom, along with his complete CV for my reference by post. I dreamed of becoming like them but without the best mentorship, research facilities and infrastructure, that dream seemed too out of reach.

On 18 May 1998, when I was at the office of the Government Medical College, Chandigarh, the fax machine buzzed. It was from Professor David J. Apple of Storm Eye Institute, Medical University of South Carolina in Charleston, USA. As I read the letter, my knees began to shake. I held the swivel chair, sat down and read slowly. 'I am pleased to offer you a research fellowship at the Centre for Research on Ocular Therapeutics and Biodevices, Storm Eye Institute, MUSC, Charleston, SC, USA for two years.' I read it again and again. I cross-checked if it was really for me. It was. I couldn't believe how far I had come. From Mohna, Jabalpur to Chandigarh, I was now about to head to the USA.

7

# Moonshot Thinking
## Landing In the USA

*'The heights by great men reached and kept were not attained by sudden flight,*
*but they, while their companions slept, were toiling upward in the night.'*
—Henry Wadsworth Longfellow

On 26 June 1998, I boarded an Air India flight from New Delhi to New York's JFK airport. It was my first international trip. My first time flying over international waters and watching India fade away into the distance. I was approaching a new world, a new life. I had called my parents a few hours before taking off. They had bid me a teary goodbye, repeating how proud they were of my accomplishments. My first pitstop was New York, from where I had a connecting flight to Charleston. But my flight reached New York two hours late.

## Charleston, Centre for IOL Research & New Challenges

The airlines put me up in a hotel and the next day, I boarded a flight to Charleston. After two hours, I was at the Charleston airport wheeling out my luggage when I saw my mentor, Professor Jagat Ram. He was there to receive me with his colleague, Dr Qun Peng. Clear blue skies welcomed me to the historical city of Charleston of South Carolina, the wealthiest and fourth largest city in colonial America, which was historically significant in both the Revolutionary and Civil Wars. The settlement, originally called Charles Towne (for Charles II), was established by English colonists in 1670 on the west bank of the Ashley River, thus beginning the colonization of South Carolina. The city moved to its present site in 1680 and became the commercial centre of trade in rice and indigo. In 1722 it was briefly incorporated as Charles City and Port, and in 1783 it was reincorporated as Charleston.

I stayed with Professor Ram that day and on the next day, 27 June 1998, Professor Ram took me to the Storm Eye Institute on what I assumed was a casual tour. We rode an elevator to the fifth floor, where sat the office of Professor David J. Apple. Professor Ram took me to the copy room, when I saw Professor Apple photocopying documents inside. He stopped midway and looked at us. He was a tall, blonde, rather handsome man. As it was a Saturday, Professor Apple was in casual wear.

I was starstruck. Professor Apple had written to me before but now here he stood before me—the founder of the Center for Developing World Ophthalmology (later renamed Centre for Research on Ocular Therapeutics and Biodevices). His laboratory served as the official collaborating centre of the Prevention of Blindness Programme of the World Health Organization (WHO). His research and meetings with WHO officials were instrumental in providing information on which type of IOL should be used in cataract surgery in developing countries. In the world of ophthalmology, Professor David J. Apple was a rockstar. The global authority on research related to intraocular lenses, ophthalmic biodevices, cataract surgery and its complications. He was called the IOL doctor's doctor. Professor Apple's Centre for Research on Ocular Therapeutics and Biodevices had a database of more than 20,000 pseudophakic human eyes (eyes implanted with an artificial lens or IOL) obtained through postmortem. His research, articles and books placed him in the hall of fame of the American Society of Cataract and Refractive Surgeons (ASCRS). Working with him was no less than a dream but even then, I had many questions: Why was their research centre so coveted? How was their research infrastructure? How did the doctors treat patients and publish so frequently? How could I maximize my learning from them?

'You must be Dr Pandey,' Professor Apple said, breaking my reverie. He had stepped forward to greet me. 'Welcome!' he said, shaking my hand. 'How was your flight?' he asked. I told him about how I missed the connecting flight and he followed up by asking me if I had slept well, if I was jetlagged, if I had eaten. It was a pleasant conversation. The following Monday, I began my journey with the Storm Eye Institute. It was my first day and I was being introduced to Professor Apple's fellows, called The Apple Korps. Professor Jagat Ram introduced me to Professor Apple's secretary, Maddie Manuel. She welcomed me with a broad smile and introduced me to other staff members. I noticed that most of them appeared happy and enthusiastic. When it was time for lunch, I decided to pull out my home-cooked Indian meal. Most senior faculty members would eat lunch at the university cafeteria or their secretaries would fix some food for them in the office, like a simple sandwich. But a few staff members and fellows brought packed lunch from home and would eat at the lunchroom. Sometimes, senior faculty members would drop in too.

I was at my desk when Professor Apple came in. 'Come, let's meet the team,' he said, and introduced me to his team members and then showed me around the lunchroom. He asked me if I had had something to eat, then enquired whether I was a vegetarian. When I told him I was, he told me so was Mahatma Gandhi. Professor Apple keenly followed the news and in May 1998, India had carried out a series of five nuclear bomb test explosions. He asked me to tell everyone about Pokhran-II. This ice-breaking conversation caused the stress within me to dissolve away. I grew at ease. After lunch, I went to the administrative office to get my ID card. The staff member, while clicking my picture, smiled and asked, 'Dr Pandey, are you happy to be here?'

'Yes,' I said.

'Then smile and let me capture your happy face!' she said.

I smiled wider and felt good about where I was. I was with people who showed me how small gestures can quell the tension. A smile, a joke, a casual reference to something that is of interest to the other person—these little gestures go a long way in dissipating nervousness and setting the foundation of friendship between people from around the world. Years later, these lessons would continue to benefit me immensely as a medical practitioner. They helped me have far superior interactions with my patients, many of whom would be tense, anxious, cynical or even suspicious.

Two days after my joining, I attended a seminar at the Storm Eye Institute auditorium, where cases were being presented by the residents. During the seminar, I met faculty members and residents of Storm Eye Institute. I still remember my first meeting with Professor M. Edward Wilson, a globally renowned paediatric ophthalmologist, became the chairman of the institute in 2000. When I saw him on the eighth floor of Storm Eye Institute, he was wheeling a teenage child around in a wheelchair. I initially thought he must be a patient or hospital attendant who wanted to bring his child in for a consultation. I later came to know that that was Professor M. Edward Wilson and it was his own son, Leland Wilson, in the wheelchair, who suffered from cerebral palsy. Professor Wilson and I have enjoyed a long, fruitful mentor–mentee relationship. He even wrote the foreword to my book, *A Hippocratic Odyssey*.* I also authored a book on paediatric

---

* Dr Suresh Pandey and Dr Vidushi Sharma, *A Hippocratic Odyssey: Lessons From a Doctor Couple on Life, In Medicine, Challenges and Doctorprneurship* (New Delhi: Bloomsbury India, 2020).

cataract surgery with him and Dr Rupal H. Trivedi,* which came to be celebrated in the ophthalmologist community.

A week later, I celebrated the US Independence Day on 4 July 1998, along with the institute staff. It felt like a personal milestone to me: a day of my freedom from relative surgical oblivion. Now that I was in the USA, I had access to many facilities that surgeons in India did not. One of the main reasons that ophthalmology residents in India were not trained well in eye microsurgery was that there were no wet lab facilities where they could practice on postmortem human eyes, model eyes or animal eyes, using the operating microscope and phacoemulsification equipment.

When I took on my first case in India, I found that performing a cataract (phacoemulsification) surgery was indeed very frightening for anyone, especially for those doing it for the first time without any prior practice in the wet lab. Any slight movement inside the eye by a novice surgeon can lead to permanent damage to the patient's cornea, or breakage of the delicate cover of the lens (known as the posterior capsule, which is only 2 to 4 micron thick in the centre and needs to be preserved for supporting any artificial implants). But at the Storm Eye Institute, I finally had the chance to perfect eye microsurgery. At the wet lab there, Professor Jagat Ram told me about the Miyake-Apple technique. This technique was first published by Dr Kensaku Miyake, a Japanese eye surgeon—I have met Dr Miyake at various ophthalmic conferences thrice and he has generously shared with me stories from his journey in ophthalmic research. Professor David Apple and his team later improved it, so it was renamed as the Miyake-Apple technique.[†]

---

* M.E. Wilson, R.H. Trivedi and S.K. Pandey, Pediatric Cataract Surgery: Techniques, Complications, and Management (Lippincott Williams & Wilkins, 2005).

† D.J. Apple, et al., 'Preparation and Study of Human Eyes Obtained Post-mortem with the Miyake Posterior Photographic Technique', Ophthalmology, 1990. DOI: https://doi.org/10.1016/S0161-6420(90)32507-.

In this technique, post-mortem human eyes are used to perform cataract surgery and study zonular stress with a high-quality camera. All novice surgeons would learn the crucial steps of cataract surgery using this technique. The research infrastructure in terms of the availability of phaco machines, operating microscopes, model eyes, post-mortem human eyes, IOLs, trephines and viscoelastic solutions was excellent, and so I began to spend most of my time learning the intricacies of eye microsurgery here.

## My Mentors and Learnings at the Mecca of IOL Research

The Storm Eye Institute was a fascinating place. One day, I saw FedEx deliver three boxes to the centre. It had small glass containers in which human eyes were carefully packed. The phakic eyes (those with natural lenses) were used for learning and practising phacoemulsification and IOL implantation. The pseudophakic eye (eye which has undergone cataract surgery and has an IOL implantation) would be used for the research purpose. Professor Apple received eyes not only from eye banks across the USA but also from eye surgeons across the world. This made learning under him the most sought-after next step for any ophthalmologist—joining the 'Apple Korps', as the international fellows under him from India, China, Europe, Brazil, Thailand, Israel, Australia, Canada etc. were called. I devoted myself to my work, staying till late on weekdays and returning on weekends. The fifth-floor Centre for Ocular Therapeutics and Biodevices was my home and a topic of amusement for my colleagues. 'Dr Pandey lives here,' they would say. Perhaps it was because of my staunch refusal to budge from making the next few years in the USA transformative for my career and giving me some of my life's most memorable moments that I spent all my time there.

Professor Apple was a delightfully positive person. He was soft-spoken and charming, and always encouraged his fellows to perform their best. He would dictate several letters using his dictaphone. He would work even while flying from place to place. We would give him our research papers before he would board the flight and he would fax us all the corrections while changing his flights. As he would be reaching his next destination, he would receive a revised manuscript from his fellows, and then we would get his inputs after a few hours. He was always happy, humble, honest and hungry for new research, which contributed greatly to his remarkable success. Each of his fellows learned many things from him. Many of them went on to become leaders.

Professor David Apple was not only adept at clinical research but also at management and delegation of tasks to those who could do them in the best possible way. I learned the art of delegation from him. Today, I delegate a lot of tasks to my capable staff. I am always connected with my patients and most of the time, my team members reply to their queries.

## New Research Partnerships

In January 1999, Dr Liliana Werner joined the institute. She came armed with stellar research experience and a PhD from Paris. We quickly developed a good working relationship. She preferred to work with me as I was very passionate about my research and would spend over ten hours a day, including weekends, working. Sometimes Dr Werner would design a study and sometimes I would do the same—write up the first draft, prepare videos and then she would read the material critically, revise it, and put in her suggestions. As per the protocol of the various projects, I would also perform surgery on rabbit eyes or human eyes obtained from postmortems.

In six months of working together, we completed three papers, the most important of which was a paper discussing the use of dye for staining mature cataracts. As most patients would wait for the cataract to mature before removing it, we wanted to find a way for doctors to overcome the barriers of performing cataract surgery in white cataract. A few years ago, a technique called phacoemulsification had started becoming popular. In this technique, an ultrasonic probe was used to break the cataractous lens nucleus into smaller pieces. But it was a challenge to perform phacoemulsification in white mature cataracts due to impaired visibility. When cataract surgery is performed using the phacoemulsification technique, one of the most important steps is creating a 5 mm circular opening at the centre of the lens capsule. This is similar to peeling the skin of potatoes after boiling them. This step is known as capsulorhexis. In immature cataracts, the red fundus reflex (seen by the surgeon through the operating microscope) is helpful in achieving the circular 5 mm central opening. In white mature cataracts (commonly seen in India), however, this red fundus glow is not seen. Therefore, staining the white mature cataract with trypan blue dyes is very helpful. Our research paper had a transformational impact upon clinical application, as most cataract cases presented in India and other developing countries tend to be at an advanced stage. The use of dye such as trypan blue can be very useful in performing successful cataract surgery on such patients.

Our research had great potential and as colleagues learnt about our work, they began to suggest how to scale it further. Professor Apple told us about the international conference called the European Society for Cataract and Refractive Surgeons (ESCRS) that was going to be held in Vienna in 1999. I decided to submit a video of me performing a surgery on postmortem human eyes and showing how trypan blue dyes could be useful to enhance visibility during cataract surgery.

## Winning the 'Oscar' of Ophthalmology

The ESCRS conference was one of the most coveted in Europe. More than 5,000 doctors, including 40 from India, were participating. The most exciting part of the conference was that on its third day, there was going to be a film festival. The jury would watch all the films submitted by doctors around the world and choose a winner. I knew I had submitted a good video but I did not think I had a chance at winning. I sat patiently in the audience, watching the programme unfold until it was time to announce the best video winner in the scientific category. 'The best video award goes to,' the host announced. I suddenly grew nervous. 'What if—' I had just begun to think when they announced, 'Dr Suresh K. Pandey'. I stood up immediately, buttoned my black suit, and walked up to the stage. The hall erupted into a roaring applause. It felt like the earth had split and taken me into another world. A world where all my hard work had paid off.

The president of ESCRS, Professor Ulf Stenevi presented me with the award and a ribbon. It was a proud moment for me when I received the prestigious film festival award at the age of thirty. *Euro Times* (the official ESCRS conference newspaper) published an interview with me. More awards followed, including the 'ASCRS Film Festival Award' by the American Society of Cataract and Refractive Surgery (ASCRS). This is popularly known as the 'Oscar' of Ophthalmology. Its jury is usually dressed in Hollywood-style black-tie, evening gowns and on the occasion, Oscar-like statues are presented to the winner. But the award was doubly special because as I stepped on stage, they played the Indian national anthem. The work of an Indian doctor was being recognized on the world stage. My heart was full.

Back at the institute, I had become the 'blue-eyed boy' of the Apple Korps. I was armed with my moonshot ambitions and never-say-never attitude. I was only just getting started.

# 8

## 'This Operation Should have Never Been Done'

### Meeting Sir Harold Ridley, The Inventor of the IOL

*'Many of life's failures are people who did not realize how close they were to success when they gave up.'*

—Thomas Alva Edison

In June 2020, as the COVID-19 pandemic raged around the world, an eighty-year-old patient came to see me in her wheelchair. She had no sight in her left eye due to twenty-year-old trauma and now her right eye had developed a cataract. She was visiting her son's family in the USA when she started developing the cataract in her right eye. Her son and daughter-in-law tried to convince her to get operated in the USA but she refused. She firmly held that cataracts should be fully mature before surgically removing them or it could lead to complications. In a few months, the cataract was fully mature and had caused a near-total vision impairment in her right eye.

Her arrival turned heads because my staff was used to seeing people from rural areas walking in with bilateral mature cataracts, but not the rich who had surgical assistance at their disposal. The cataract had matured within three months and I was certain that cataract surgery and artificial intraocular lens implantation were the only solution. The patient had corneal astigmatism or uneven curvature of the cornea, which blurred and distorted her vision. But she did not want to wear glasses. A person who has both cataract and corneal astigmatism cannot regain quality distance vision after cataract surgery unless the astigmatism is also corrected. This meant that I would have to use the uniquely-designed intraocular lenses in the only eye that could be salvaged. The patient's son and daughter-in-law were somewhat distrustful of Indian doctors. But they relented at their mother's insistence. The surgery was challenging not only because of the dense cataract but also because of the patient's one-eye status.

I first used a diamond blade to make a tiny 2.8 mm wide incision in her peripheral cornea to enter the eye. Then I inserted a Malyugin ring (invented by Russian eye surgeon Dr Boris Malyugin), a square-shaped transitory implant, whose four circular loops grasp the iris and dilate the pupil. I took out a small needle with a bent tip to make a circular hole in the lens capsule. This felt as if I were peeling an orange zest. An ultrasonic probe connected to a phacoemulsification machine was then inserted in the hole of the crystalline lens of the eye. Once activated, it broke and sucked out the nucleus and cortex of the cataract. Then with a deep breath and steady hands, I injected a folded artificial intraocular lens into the eye through a 2.8 mm incision. I watched with satisfaction as it unfolded and positioned itself on the lens capsule. The surgery was successfully completed and she was thrilled to regain her vision after a 15-minute surgery without a single injection, stitch or pain.

## Royal Air Force, Rayner and Ridley's First Intraocular Lens

The Age-related cataract remains the most common cause of blindness around the world. Cataract surgery along with the implantation of an artificial intraocular lens (IOL) is the most commonly performed surgery on the human body. Yet, many are unaware of the invention of IOL that has helped millions regain their vision. It's a story zealously guarded by ophthalmologists but clouded from public consciousness and forgotten over time. It's the story of Dr Harold Ridley, a quiet, unassuming doctor from London, and Lieutenant Gordon Mouse Cleaver, a Royal Air Force pilot.

Mouse Cleaver was a member of the No. 601 Squadron, informally called the Millionaires' Squadron because its pilots were former elite British sportsmen. They flew Hawker Hurricanes, the fighter aircraft especially designed for World War II. In France in 1940, Cleaver claimed a Dornier Do 17, Nazi Germany's flight bomber, and clinched his first victory. Then he was sent back to England to fight the Battle of Britain. On 15 August 1940, Cleaver had to fly a few sorties. He did so and met his unit for lunch. He was quickly ordered to return when, in haste, he forgot his safety goggles. He was flying somewhere over the city of Winchester and was lined up behind the Junkers Ju 88, a German combat aircraft, when machine-gun fire raked his aircraft. His airplane burst into flames. He flipped the aircraft upside down and jumped out of the cockpit. Mid-air, he opened his parachute and landed on the ground. But he wasn't safe. Acrylic shards from the aircraft's canopy were lodged in his eyes. His right eye was severely damaged and couldn't be saved. Dr Ridley examined him and directed all his attention to the left eye. Cleaver underwent eighteen operations to treat his facial wounds and restore some vision in his left eye. When a squadron friend came to see him, Cleaver said, 'Tell them to wear their goggles'. But Cleaver's fate helped Dr Ridley make an astonishing discovery.

Dr Ridley was nagged by a certain peculiarity of Cleaver's case: other than damaging the lens, the plastic splinters in Cleaver's left eye did not affect his sight, nor did his body reject them. He mused if he could use a plastic lens to replace the natural one removed during cataract surgery. This thought was reinforced one day in 1948 when

Stephen Perry, a medical student, watched Dr Ridley operate. 'Dr Ridley,' Perry commented innocuously, 'it is a pity you cannot replace the cataract with a clear lens.' The words might have been wishful but they sparked an idea in Dr Ridley's mind. He remembered the plastic splinters in Cleaver's eyes and wondered if it would be possible to make an artificial lens of the same material and insert it into the eyes. Dr Ridley was daring to go against the accepted norms of ophthalmology, which was all about removing things from the eye, not putting anything in. He knew how conservative his fellow doctors could be and he decided that if he had to do something, he had to do it as secretly as possible. He reached out to John Pike, a scientist he knew at Rayner and Keeler Ltd., a prominent British optical company, and invited to meet him in his car parked outside a public park. Dr Ridley tasked the manufacturer with building the first artificial intraocular lens. It was biconvex, like the natural lens, with an equatorial ridge that could be used to grasp and handle it using surgical instruments. The Ridley IOL was different from the modern-day IOL. It did not contain the IOL haptics—two long C loops known as haptics are helpful to ensure the correct placement of the lens.

A few months after the lens was readied, Dr Ridley identified the first patient to receive the implant. It was a wintry day on 29 November 1949. At St. Thomas Hospital, London, wind from the Thames was making the windows chatter. Inside the operation theatre, masked and gloved surgeons performed a surgery in secret. After removing the cataract, Dr Ridley inserted the artificial IOL but as soon as he had done it, he suddenly wavered. He was not sure if it would stay in place. He decided to remove the IOL and close the eye. Perhaps, he thought, after the postoperative inflammation had healed, he could insert it again. Two months later, on 8 February 1950, he performed the second surgery, which succeeded. Soon, Dr Ridley performed ten such operations. All were successful. The eye took in the lens and tolerated it pretty well. Dr Ridley also learnt that the lens' power had to be adjusted because the refractive power of the lens in the aqueous fluid of the eye was different from its power in the open air.

But Dr Ridley stayed put. He did not publish or share the results of his surgeries for two years. He wanted to create a watertight case for the use of IOLs through a series of patients. But the news of his stunning discovery leaked in the most anti-climactic way. One of Dr Harold Ridley's patients skimmed through the phonebook to make a new appointment with him. He found Dr Frederick Ridley, another ophthalmologist in London, and mistook him for the doctor who had operated on him. The patient went to the appointment, was examined by the other Dr Ridley, and the secret was revealed. Dr Ridley received the news, deadpan. He sped up the completion of his articles and decided to go public himself. The word spread like wildfire. Everyone was talking about eyes and lenses.

The response was unfavourable. Dr Ridley's fellow doctors accused him of malpractice. They excoriated him for the complications, which included corneal edema, glaucoma and IOL dislocation. What about theoretical complications, they argued, such as sympathetic ophthalmia, a severe autoimmune reaction that affects the fellow eye, and even malignancy? Dr Ridley was surrounded by condemnation and criticism. He was deeply disturbed, afraid of being sued or losing his hospital privileges.

But progressive ophthalmologists showed support. Eye doctors with an interest in IOL implants formed the International Intraocular Implant Club (IIIC). The club was founded in 1966 by the English ophthalmic surgeons Sir Harold Ridley and Peter Choyce to promote research in the field of intraocular lens implantation. At that time, there was widespread opposition to the use of IOLs. I was very fortunate to become a member of the prestigious IIIC in 2002. I was perhaps the youngest Indian to get the membership of this historical club at the age of thirty-four. The aim of IIIC was to promote IOL research, reduce implant-related complications and improve outcomes. This acceptance of IOL gradually grew more and more. It epitomized what Victor Hugo once wrote, 'Nothing is more powerful than an idea whose time has come'.

In 1989 and 1990, Dr Ridley himself developed cataract and received IOL implantation to regain 6/6 vision in each eye. Now, IOL is widely accepted and a standard feature of quality care. But it wasn't good enough. Dr Ridley frequently brought to light that the resistance to his ideas delayed the cure of aphakia or the absence of lens in the eye for twenty-five years. This meant that an entire generation of cataract patients needlessly suffered aphakia, or a condition in which the lens is absent. Dr Ridley did not patent his IOL. He believed the invention belonged to everyone. Indeed, since 1950, 8 million cataract surgeries with IOL implantation have been performed around the world. They are a direct result of Dr Ridley's efforts. After years of resistance, the world honoured him unequivocally.*

Today, IOLs are so advanced that they can be folded to fit through a 1.8 mm incision and then open inside the eye as they are guided into position. Presbyopia-correcting IOLs permit patients to see both near, intermediate and far. Phakic refractive IOLs are implanted into the healthy eyes of young people who have high-refractive error (high myopia) as an alternative to refractive surgery. The treatment for cataracts had not progressed one iota for centuries. In just the last thirty years, however, it has advanced rapidly.

In 1988, I was glancing over an ophthalmic newsletter *Ocular Surgery News* during my posting in the department of ophthalmology at NSCB Medical College, Jabalpur. A news item announced that Flight Lieutenant Mouse Cleaver's left eye had been implanted with an intraocular lens and he had regained his eyesight. By then I was a third-year medical student. I picked up the tabloid and read closely.

---

* He was knighted by Queen Elizabeth II on 9 February 2000. He was 93 and lived to see his efforts recognized. He died the next year. In 2003, two stamps honouring him were issued by the British Postal Service.

The words intraocular lens seemed alien, unknown. Who was Dr Harold Ridley? I didn't know that in the years to come, I would work with his invention almost every day of my life. Or that twelve years later, I would have breakfast with him.

\* \* \*

In May 2000, I was in Boston for an eye conference. At that time, I was working with Professor David Apple, who had invited Dr Harold Ridley and his wife Elizabeth to the conference. I was a bag of nerves. Shaking and trembling, I got up on the dais and spoke about the impact of IOL in India, especially in the lives of children. I thanked Dr Ridley for bringing light and vision to their lives. I felt happy and fulfilled, even though I hadn't yet had a chance to talk to him personally.

On the last day, as I arrived at the hotel's restaurant for breakfast, I saw Dr Ridley and his wife at one of the tables. I approached them and Dr Ridley recognized me. 'Dr Pandey from India,' he said. I beamed. He told me how his wife was born in Nainital as I settled down next to them. For several minutes, I listened to Dr Ridley talk about the journey of his incredible life. I was starry-eyed and in awe. I couldn't believe that I had reached where I was. As I looked at the affable face of Dr Ridley and his wife, I thought back to my own life—my grandfather who had ignited my passion, my early education and my village from where I rose to reach the United States of America.

# 9

# Collaborating and Learning from Peers

*'Alone we can do so little; together we can do so much.'*

—Helen Keller

It had been eighteen months since my last visit to India. As 1999 came to an end, I decided to make another short trip back home. I boarded a Delta Airlines flight and reached New Delhi on the cold night of 30 December 1999. From New Delhi, I went to Chandigarh and celebrated New Year's there with my old friends. It was a grand homecoming. The next day, I met Professor Amod Gupta, Professor Jagat Ram, Professor Mangat R. Dogra and other faculty members. I wanted to express my gratitude to them for their perseverance in teaching and training new residents like me. Most of the faculty members knew about my publications in prestigious international journals and the awards I had received.

As I bowed to touch their feet, Professor Amod Gupta, Professor Jagat Ram and Professor Mangat R. Dogra congratulated me and said, 'Well done, Dr Pandey. We are very proud of you.' I felt like my life's hard work had paid off. My teachers were happy with the work I had done. Then my life came full circle: Professor Amod Gupta, chief of the eye department at that time, invited me to deliver a guest lecture at the Department of Ophthalmology, PGIMER, Chandigarh. It was an unexpected request but it gratified me deeply. I presented the work on my research on dye-enhanced cataract surgery, IOL opacification, piggyback IOLs and others. There was a question-answer session where I answered the questions of the faculty members and residents. It was a proud moment to deliver a lecture in the same lecture room where I once sat as a student.

I then travelled home to meet my parents in Kota, where I got a hero's welcome. They were very happy to know what I was doing, especially my father, for whom I had fulfilled his life's dream. After a few days, I took their blessings and left for Chennai. Dr Jyotirmay Biswas (chief of the uveitis unit) invited me to deliver a guest lecture at the Sankara Nethralaya. Once again, this was a place that I had aspired to visit and work at. And here I was, delivering a talk there. I thought back to my time in the USA and before that at PGIMER, Chandigarh, and realized that one reason why I had managed to do what I did was through the power of collaboration.

## Pioneering Research on Piggyback IOLs or Polypseudophakia

It was November 1999 and I was in the USA Thanksgiving Day was around the corner and the country was abuzz with preparations. One morning, Professor Apple called me to his office and gave me a letter and a pair of explanted IOLs for research and evaluation. The pair had been submitted to Professor Apple's lab by a renowned eye surgeon, Dr Johnny L. Gayton.

Sir Harold Ridley had invented the single IOL but Dr Johnny Gayton had invented the technique of implanting two intraocular lenses in the eye. He called this technique 'Piggyback IOL' or 'Polypseudophakia'.* It was particularly useful for patients whose

---

* J.L. Gayton, V. Sanders, et al., 'Piggybacking intraocular implants to correct pseudophakic refractive error', *Ophthalmology*, 106, 1999, pp. 56–59.

eye refractive power was high. Back then, most IOL manufacturers did not manufacture IOLs beyond 30 dioptres. Dr Gayton had a solution: since the 40 Dioptre IOL was not manufactured, he implanted two IOLs of 20 Dioptre each in the eye. The patient did well for two years but after that, his vision decreased. That's when Dr Gayton approached Professor Apple and I was assigned to help him. Until this moment, I had believed that success meant being at the right place, at the right time. But I realized that people miss an important attribute: the right company. Not only was I at the right place, at the right time, but I was also among people who believed in teamwork and collaboration.

When the patient arrived, Dr Gayton carefully examined his left eye. He found that there was a membrane between the two lenses. Both IOLs (with membrane) were explanted from the eye by Dr Gayton and he submitted detailed evaluations. Then it was my turn to observe him. After examining the explanted IOLs, I saw that it was this membrane that was causing opacity between these two IOLs. We saw that two IOLs were stuck to each other and documented the presence of this membrane. We termed it as interlenticular opacification (ILO). This was followed by extensive research and observations. We found that different surgical methods could prevent this complication.

I was encouraged by Dr Gayton's enthusiasm to work on this research and was ecstatic at the learning opportunity. We shot a video on our findings and sent it out to international conferences and seminars. Wherever the video went, it won awards. Our research, too, was published in top ophthalmology journals that include the *American Journal of Ophthalmology*, *Archives of Ophthalmology* and *Journal of Cataract and Refractive Surgery*.* This collaboration with a global leader in ophthalmology not only gave me a chance to learn, but also helped

---

* S.K. Pandey, M.E. Snyder, et al., 'Interlenticular opacification (ILO): Clinical and pathological lessons for prevention and management', (prize- winning video); S.K. Pandey, L. Werner, et al., 'Interlenticular opacification after piggyback intraocular lens

me produce several award-winning videos and scientific publications for top peer-reviewed ophthalmic journals. It reaffirmed my faith in working collaboratively, with support and sensitivity towards your team members.

## Cataract of the Artificial Lens: IOL Opacification

Another collaborative opportunity came in the form of a cataract of the IOL. During the late 1990s, many patients implanted with an IOL complained of blurry and faded vision. Doctors were in a fix. What was going wrong? Few doctors thought this could be what is called the posterior capsule opacification (after cataract) and tried to create an opening using a YAG laser. One such case of opacified IOL visited Dr Mahmut Kaskaloglu in Turkey. He decided to remove the IOL from the eye and send it to Professor Apple's lab. I was assigned the case. When I researched, I found that opacification of the IOL was due to the deposition of calcium. This was a path-breaking finding with immediate repercussions.

Based on our research and publications, many leading manufacturers started creating the IOL from hydrophobic acrylic material instead of the formerly used hydrophilic acrylic. I was in the USA, in the cradle of world-changing innovation and I got the opportunity to collaborate with several other globally renowned ophthalmologists like Dr Richard J. Linnola from Finland, Dr Beatrice Cochener from France, Dr Anthony J. Maloof from Australia, Dr Abhay R. Vasavada, Dr Amar Agarwal, Dr Natarajan Sundaram

implantation' won the 'Best Cataract' poster, presented at the ASCRS Symposium on Cataract, IOL and Refractive Surgery, April–May 2001, San Diego, CA, USA).

L. Werner, D.J. Apple et al., 'Analysis of elements of interlenticular opacification', *American Journal of Ophthalmology*, 133(3), March 2002, pp.: 320–6. doi: 10.1016/s0002-9394(01)01405-2. PMID: 11860967.

And D.J. Apple, L. Werner, S.K. Pandey, 'Newly recognized complications of posterior chamber intraocular lenses', *Arch Ophthalmol*, 119(4), April 2001, pp.: 581–2. doi: 10.1001/archopht.119.4.581. PMID: 11296025.

and Dr Mahipal Singh Sachdev from India. Each collaboration was special, widened my understanding of ophthalmology and helped me position myself as a leading practitioner. After the many dark days of my childhood, I was now looking towards the light. My future was bright.

## Collaborations in India

Dr Abhay R. Vasavada was the first globally renowned Indian ophthalmologist who inspired me the most. For the first time, I watched him demonstrating the 'Live Phaco Surgery' at Sadguru Netra Chikitsalaya, Chitrakoot, in 1993 during the Madhya Pradesh State Ophthalmology Society conference. His elegant way of speaking and artistic way of demonstrating, explaining, teaching each and every minute step in surgery in detail, impressed me the most. Later on, I assisted him in performing live surgery at PGIMER, Chandigarh, during the All India Ophthalmology Society (AIOS) Conference in 1996. Dr Abhay R. Vasavada and I collaborated on a few research projects in the USA and also participated in several instruction courses at ASCRS, ESCRS and the AAO conference. We also published papers in prestigious ophthalmology journals. Dr Vasavada visited Kota during the Rajasthan Ophthalmological Society (ROS) Conference held in 2008 and the newly established SuVi Eye Hospital, Kota.

I also had the opportunity to work with another world-renowned Indian eye surgeon, Dr Amar Agarwal, on several research projects like no-anaesthesia cataract surgery, or phakonit or cataract surgery through a 0.9 mm incision. This research was published in the prestigious American ophthalmology journal, *The Journal of Cataract and Refractive Surgery.*[*] I also authored thirty book chapters and edited

---

[*] S.K. Pandey, M.D. Agarwal et al., 'No-Anesthesia Versus Topical and Topical Plus Intracameral Anesthesia', *Journal of Cataract & Refractive Surgery*, 28(7), July 2002, p. 1087. DOI: 10.1016/S0886-3350(02)01471-2.

six books in association with him. I also had the opportunity to stay at his house during the Intraocular Implant & Refractive Society, India (IIRSI) conference in Chennai in 2000, where I was honoured with a gold medal. Working with Dr Amar Agarwal gave me a keen insight into his passion and his work schedule. He would sleep only five hours, 9.30 P.M. to 2.30 A.M., and would often reply to my emails in the dead of night. Every week, he would travel to deliver talks and lectures and almost every year, he would introduce new innovative techniques. He was and remains one of the most efficient, multitasking go-getters I know. Watching him has helped me improve my own energy and efficiency.

I also had the opportunity to collaborate with another efficient, energetic eye surgeon, Padma Shri Professor Natarajan Sundaram, fondly called 'Nutty' by his friends. 7 April is celebrated as World Health Day. This is a special day for us as it is my wife, Dr Vidushi's birthday as well. Every year, she would deliver a lecture on the occasion of World Health Day at the programme organized by the Indian Medical Association, Kota. I was working as secretary of IMA Kota during the year 2016 and we invited Padma Shri Dr Natarajan Sundaram to deliver the prestigious World Health Day lecture. We also planned a programme to inaugurate the DORC Eva Machine. This machine was the first in all of Rajasthan and Madhya Pradesh, and only the second to be installed in India. Dr Natarajan inaugurated the DORC Eva machine on 7 April 2016. This was combined with Dr Vidushi's birthday celebrations. In the evening, he presented the World Health Day oration at the IMA House, Kota. Everyone appreciated Dr Natarajan's work in the field of diabetic retinopathy and his commendable work in Mumbai's Dharavi slums.

I had known Dr Natarajan Sundaram since my days in PGIMER, Chandigarh in 1995. I participated in and chaired a session with him during the Asia Pacific Academy of Cataract and Refractive Surgery (APACRS) conference in Shanghai in 2013. He is always smiling and full of energy. He travelled around the world to present papers or perform live surgeries. His presentations were not only related to ophthalmology—he spoke on several subjects including how to increase efficiency, energy, happiness and positivity. Most of my ophthalmologist colleagues would joke that everyone is a regular Eveready battery and he is a Duracell Energizer battery. His untiring energy and stamina even at the age of sixty-six continues to inspire me.

## Live Surgery: A Fifteen-Year Dream Comes True

I had the opportunity to collaborate with a great ophthalmic entrepreneur, Padma Shri Dr Mahipal Singh Sachdev, for the first time when I was a resident at PGIMER, Chandigarh, in 1996. He performed a live surgery at the operation theatre there. I was standing near him as one of his assistants and dreaming that one day I too would get the chance to perform a live surgery. Nearly fifteen years later, in 2010, I had the opportunity to do so alongside him twice at the Centre for Sight, New Delhi, during the Delhi Ophthalmology Society (DOS) Conference. After that, I had the chance to perform twenty-five live surgeries in New Delhi, Chennai, Chandigarh, Pune, Hyderabad, Vizag, Ahmedabad, Vadodara, Mumbai, Jaipur, Jodhpur, Udaipur, Alwar, Kota, etc. Dr Sachdev was a teacher of Dr Vidushi's at AIIMS, New Delhi, and a famous entrepreneur who established the Centre for Sight in 1986, which today has more than fifty branches in India and ten abroad.

Dr Ritika Sachdev, his daughter, visited Kota in May 2016 during one of the Continued Medical Education (CME) programs. During conversation, she told us that ophthalmologists had gained much recognition, respect and remuneration during the past two decades. She told us about an incident when her father was getting married to her mother, Dr Alka Sachdev, a gynaecologist. Dr Alka's parents were worried about Dr Mahipal's future financial status but with the robust growth of the Centre for Sight, Dr Mahipal attracted funding from big financers, including Mahindra and Mahindra.

During the past ten years, Indian ophthalmology has progressed by leaps and bounds. The All India Ophthalmological Society became the largest ophthalmology society in the world with the maximum life members (25,000). I continue to be inspired by the youngest, talented Indian eye surgeons and by the Indian ophthalmology gurus and observe very closely their strengths and the qualities that make them different. I often thought our country would become the global leader in ophthalmology. After all, India has a hundred leaders like Dr Amod Gupta, Dr Jagat Ram, Dr Abhay R. Vasavada, Dr Amar Agarwal, Dr Mahipal S. Sachdev, Dr Jeewan S. Titiyal, Dr Natarajan Sundaram, Dr Santosh G. Honavar, Dr Sri Ganesh, Dr Rohit Shetty, etc. Indian women ophthalmologists like Dr Namatra Sharma, Dr Soosan Jacob, etc. made it to the list of the top 100 influential ophthalmologists worldwide. I am sure that Indian ophthalmology is on its path to acquiring global leadership in the next ten to fifteen years.

* * *

Working with leaders of ophthalmology from around the world has taught me a lot. But I often wonder how I can distil this information for the benefit of others. One thing they all have in common is what Eleanor Roosevelt once said, 'A good leader inspires people to have confidence in the leader, a great leader inspires people to have confidence in themselves'. Successful leaders know how to assemble a dedicated and efficient team. They're also excellent communicators and in fact, they tend to over-communicate because they don't make assumptions. They pay attention to being authentic and reliable. They're themselves. They don't pretend in order to be liked. In fact, they align their work with their values. They also face obstacles with courage and never allow themselves to feel demotivated by them.

And perhaps most importantly, successful leaders stay calm even during the most stressful times. As I made a note of these qualities in my diary, I thought I was only doing it for myself and for the expansion of my own understanding. I didn't know that very soon, I would be turning the pages of this diary again, not in the pursuit of knowledge but to find inspiration for my own entrepreneurial venture.

# 10

# Towards a Fulfilling Life

## Marriage and Beyond

*'If one advances confidently in the direction of his dreams and endeavours to live the life he has imagined, he will meet with a success unexpected in common hours.'*

—Henry David Thoreau

I flew from Charleston to Philadelphia to participate in the ASCRS Conference from 1–5 June 2002. On 1 June 2002, I woke up to the news of a conflict on the Indo-Pak border. It typically would have had little bearing on my life. Many civilians live divorced from the realities of conflicted regions. But this time I wasn't as sure. Two years ago, India and Pakistan had fought the Kargil War and rumours of another armed conflict were rife. Just before this escalation on the border, there had been a huge development in my life. My elder sister's matrimonial advertisement for me in the *Times of India* had got a response after seven days. I got a call from Group Captain Indian Air Force K.M. Sharma in January 2002 on my USA number. After exchanging pleasantries, he expressed his desire to meet my parents. I didn't object. After this conversation, I called him once a month. I also began an email correspondence with his daughter Dr Vidushi, who I thought was the perfect combination of simplicity and brilliance.

Group Capt. Sharma suggested that I plan to visit India. I looked at my calendar and decided that I could pay a visit six months later, in June 2002. I had been in the USA for four years and thought that perhaps it was time for me to find a life partner. But the news of the escalating border conflict dissuaded me. I gathered my thoughts and spoke to Group Capt Sharma. 'Maybe I should postpone my visit,' I suggested and heard an uproarious laughter from his end. 'This is nothing,' he said. 'Mere *Gidarbhabki*, cowardice from Pakistan.'

His confidence calmed me. I decided to make the trip. I landed in India on 13 June 2002 and Group Capt. Sharma came to receive me at the airport. He drove us to their Noida home. It was about 8 A.M. I was tired after a long flight but when Dr Vidushi offered me some coffee, I immediately felt refreshed. She looked beautiful in a blue salwar kurta. After a while, her parents left us alone to talk and we had detailed conversations about politics, life in Kota and the USA.

## Pandey Ji Poori and Pakora Wale

Dr Vidushi asked me about my life in the USA and if I cooked my meals on my own. She also asked me what my favourite dish was. I told her that I could cook Indian food and I am considered as a 'poori and pakora expert' by my colleagues and friends in the USA. I was living in an apartment close to the Medical University of South Carolina campus in Charleston. More than twenty researchers from India were in the building. Every Sunday morning, we would gather to cook and hold a *satsang* at one of the apartments. A few Americans would also attend and I was surprised to note that they had turned completely vegetarian and followed the Hindu teachings with unmoving faith. For these get-togethers, I would cook pooris and pakoras. Gradually, my cooking skills got better and better, and I was able to prepare food for twenty–thirty people with ease. I was appreciated by my colleagues and they fondly called me 'Pandey Ji Poori and Pakora wale'. Some of them even suggested I start a food stall chain by the same name.

Dr Vidushi still tells our close friends how after our wedding in June 2002, she and I moved to Sydney, where she cooked and I did the dishes and cleaned the kitchen. This gave me an opportunity to truly become a 'cooking and cleaning expert'.

It was obvious that Dr Vidushi's parents were deeply appreciative of my journey. Group Capt. Sharma had risen through the ranks after working his way out of his village in Kasison, Aligarh, UP. Perhaps he saw a little bit of himself in me. But I didn't know how Dr Vidushi felt until much later, when she told me that she liked that I was down-to-earth person and not an 'MCP'. I asked her who or what an 'MCP' was. She explained to me that MCP was short for 'male chauvinist pig', or a man who thought himself superior because of his gender and barked orders at his wife at home. I told her about what I had coined as a 'miserable male child syndrome', wherein the male children of the house do nothing—not even make tea—and are pitifully dependent on the women for everything. I had similar views as her on gender discrimination.

I didn't think that I was superior because I was born a boy. This was because of a range of factors. One, unlike many young boys, I grew up around girls and women. My parents never discriminated between my sister and us brothers. My elder sister, Usha Pandey, took up a government job and supported the family just like a son would. My medical college batch had fifty girls and ninety boys. Since I was polite, had no airs and was happy to be of any help to anyone, few female classmates would approach me for work and I would do it without any hesitation. Second, I grew up reading books and magazines, especially a spiritual magazine, *Akhand Jyoti*. The author, Gurudev Pandit Shri Ram Sharma Acharya, wrote that the reason India was lagging behind was because we have not given opportunities to our women.

One day in June 1986, I visited Shantikunj Ashram in Haridwar. Vandniya Mataji (wife of Gurudev Pandit Shri Ram Sharma Acharya) was addressing the gathering of devotees, saying that Guruji had never even asked her for a glass of water. He had always motivated her to lead the mission of Gayatri Pariwar. Teachings like this had a huge impact on my mind.

Ten days after this, Dr Vidushi and I got married. I was thrilled to be with someone like her who was not only exceptionally qualified in her work, but also a kind human being. Having a doctor partner also solidified my desire to build a hospital in North India. But I still needed more experience. I dreamt of becoming the finest eye surgeon in the world and for that, I needed exposure.

## Sydney, Surgical Fellowship and a Shared Dream

I applied and got through a surgical (anterior segment) fellowship in Australia. Dr Vidushi applied too and was selected for an oculoplastic fellowship at Sydney Eye Hospital under the mentorship of Professor Peter Martin and Professor Ross S. Benger. I moved to Australia in December 2002 and Dr Vidushi joined the fellowship in January 2003. We rented an apartment and started our life in Sydney. We lived in Darlinghurst, in the heart of the city. It was a charming neighbourhood with trendy cafés, a prestigious medical corridor, world-class museums and prestigious private schools. Over the weekends, we began to explore Sydney's waterfront and skyscrapers.

We visited the Sydney Opera House, Darling Harbour, the arched Harbour Bridge and the esteemed Royal Botanic Garden nearby. We also visited Sydney Tower's outdoor platform, the Skywalk, which offers stunning 360-degree views of the city and its suburbs. In March 2003, we saw the largest Sydney Gay and Lesbian Mardi Gras. It was spellbinding to be part of one of Australia's biggest tourist attractions, with the parade and dance party attracting many international and domestic tourists. All along, Dr Vidushi and I were getting to know each other. We realized that as doctors, we were similar—bound by ethics and committed to give our best efforts for patient satisfaction. In every other aspect, we balanced each other out. I was a driven and motivated researcher, she was more composed and relaxed. I was an average writer and speaker, whereas Dr Vidushi was excellent in these aspects. We completed each other, both at home and work.

My mentor at the Intraocular Implant Unit, Sydney Eye Hospital, Dr E. John Milverton, was an ambidextrous surgeon. I was a left-handed surgeon. He motivated me to start practising using my right, non-dominant hand. He suggested that I start by using it to brush my teeth, draw shapes like circles and triangles. I followed his advice religiously and eventually became an ambidextrous surgeon myself.

In 2004, I was close to finishing my fellowship in Sydney, but I continued to spend erratic working hours in the office. Meanwhile, from 2003–2004, Dr Vidushi was working with Professor Peter Martin and Professor Ross S. Benger, both world-renowned oculoplastic surgeons. She was conducting innovative research on dacryo-cysto-rhinostomy (DCR) surgery which was published in the *American Journal of Ophthalmology*.* For another year, Dr Vidushi worked with Professor Frank A. Billson in the paediatric ophthalmology department. Professor Billson had the same working style as me. I spent many nights at the office and so did he. He was then one of the most experienced, well-known and well-respected doctors in the world, and I believed I was in good company. He would work at his office from 10 P.M. to 4 A.M. on the weekends, while I would be in the adjoining room, writing my book on paediatric cataract surgery.

---

* V. Sharma et al., 'Evaluation of the cosmetic significance of external dacryocystorhinostomy scars', Am J Ophthalmol, 140(3), 2005, pp. 359–62. doi: 10.1016/j.ajo.2005.04.039. PMID: 16083840.

In the middle of the night, Professor Billson and I would take a break and meet for coffee. I taught him the art of phaco surgery in the wet lab and so we got to spend a lot of time together. Professor Billson was very friendly with all students, residents and fellows. He offered me his inputs for my book. I included his input, after which the book was published with both our names on it.

On one such day in November, as we sipped coffee, he asked me what I thought of pursuing an academic career in Australia. I asked him how I could stay in Australia and get the Royal Australian and New Zealand College of Ophthalmology (RANZCO) accreditation without appearing for the examination. After finishing his coffee, he wrote on a tissue paper: 'It will depend on creating a perception about you'.

'Dr Pandey,' he said, 'you have an excellent academic record. We would be happy to appoint you as an associate professor in the department of ophthalmology.' I couldn't believe my ears. I told Professor Billson that it was a great plan. But once again, I found myself at a crossroads—I wanted to return to India, but also knew that the opportunity in Sydney was unmatchable. So Dr Vidushi and I made another life-changing decision at that stage. I looked back at my career. Nobody's career follows an upward graph all the time and medicine is no different. In India, more than 20.8 lakh NEET aspirants appeared in 2023,[*] hoping to get into a good medical college, thinking that success in that one examination was their ticket to a career that would rise and rise. The exam does indeed provide you with a direction, but there are many challenges after that. The trials that follow may not seem as daunting as clearing the exam, but they are trials nonetheless.

Professor Billson was very keen that we stay in Sydney. On one November evening, he invited us to dinner at his residence, where

---

[*] Manash Pratim Gohain, 'Over 20 lakh applicants for NEET UG 2023', *Times of India*, 20 April 2023. Available at: https://timesofindia.indiatimes.com/education/news/over-20-lakh-applicants-for-neet-ug-2023/articleshow/99621365.cms

his wife, Gail, told us about her visit to India and Professor Billson tried to convince us of the bright future we could have in Australia. Dr Vidushi and I took several weeks to make up our minds. We had become doctors because we wanted to enter a noble and respected profession that could make a difference in people's lives. That difference may be something as big as saving a life, providing the gift of sight, or it may be something as small as helping to relieve somebody's pain. I also became a doctor to honour my first hero, my grandfather, and to walk in his footsteps to help the needy.

Still, we had got used to the comfortable life in Sydney. How could we leave such a beautiful city, turn down such a lucrative offer and move back to India? It was one of the most difficult decisions for us to make. Then finally, it came down to our long-term ambitions in life. And there we found two common grounds: first was to help eliminate preventable blindness, and the second was enlightening young medical students. According to WHO, India is now home to the world's largest number of blind people. Every third blind person is an Indian. Of the 39 million people across the globe who are blind, over 15 million are from India. What's worse, 75 per cent of these are cases of avoidable blindness due to the acute shortage of ophthalmologists, optometrists and donated eyes for the treatment of corneal blindness in the country. While India needs 50,000 optometrists, it has only 11,000; it needs 2.5 lakh donated eyes every year but the country's 109 eye banks manage to collect a maximum of just 25,000 eyes, 30 per cent of which can't be used. India has more than 23,000 ophthalmologists—too few to tackle the huge burden of treating preventable blindness.* During the past seventeen years, we have successfully performed more than 1 lakh sight-restoring eye surgeries. Blindness can be eradicated from India, provided each and every eye surgeon is fully committed to working for the same with complete dedication.

---

* 'Towards Developing India Eye Health Action Plan', VISION 2020, 2015.

In addition to this, we both wanted to motivate young medical students to get the best exposure and opportunities. I had risen from very humble beginnings. We had both received the best possible ophthalmic surgical training in India and overseas. And now, it was time that we paid it back to our own people. This was how we could encourage young doctors to continue to provide good service in their home country.

# 11

# The Accidental Entrepreneur

## Coming Back to India

*'What lies behind us and what lies before us are tiny matters compared to what lies within us.'*

—Walt Emerson

In early 2005, Dr Vidushi and I decided to return to India. We called it a bold move but many others thought it was heedless. They were not wrong. We had decided that before setting up our own hospital, we would gain some experience at an established healthcare facility in India. Joining a prestigious institute as faculty members seemed like a viable option. Just a few days before moving, we met our prospective boss at the RANZCO conference in Hobart, Australia. He asked me to call him by his first name. I thought, wow, he must be the friendliest boss. But when the time for a serious discussion came, things went awry. He told me that out of five days a week, one day would be to run clinics, another for the operation theatre, and the other four days were marked for research. But this wasn't pure research.

During this time, Dr Vidushi and I were also expected to apply for research grants and get as much funding as possible from governments, private institutions and my contacts in the USA. 'We are training a lot of eye surgeons and getting eye surgeons a dime a dozen,' he told me. Not only was he offering us a low salary, he also tried to drill into my head that my real job was to win research grants and funding.

I found this offer highly unappealing. Somehow, after talking to him, we realized that nothing about the job worked for us: neither the salary nor the limitations on clinico-surgical work. We declined his offer and decided to go back to the drawing board. We were leaving for India in two weeks but had no idea what we wanted to do there. All we knew was that we had vague entrepreneurial ambitions of setting up our own medical practice and eye hospital. We thought that perhaps, we could make it work. As writer Mark Manson says, 'Improving our lives hinges not on our ability to turn lemons into lemonade, but on learning to stomach lemons better'.

## The Long Way Back Home

India currently has around 15 million blind people against 39 million globally, which makes India home to one-third of the world's blind population. The total number of eye surgeons in India is only 23,000 to deal with 1.2 billion plus population. Many doctors leave India after completing their education. I read about how Dr Gullapalli N. Rao returned to India and established the L.V. Prasad Eye Institute in Hyderabad. You can imagine if Dr Rao had not returned to India, what a loss it would have been for our country.

My father-in-law, now retired Group Capt. K.M. Sharma, also encouraged me to return to India. He said, 'Be your own boss in India. It is better to be a king in Hell rather than a servant in Heaven'. In addition to professional reasons, I came back to India for the same reason you go back home at the end of the day—it is home and it feels like home. So many people asked me whether one should stay abroad or come back to India. There is no right or wrong answer, I believe. I think people should do whatever makes them comfortable and wherever they see better opportunities for growth.

When I was doing my fellowship, everyone would ask me what my plans were, and when I said I would go back to India after a few years, most would find it hard to believe. They would say, 'I will ask you this question after five years when you still are in the US.' But I returned to India. I don't understand what the big deal is. The US is a very nice place in many respects, but there are advantages and disadvantages to living in every country.

Even though I came back to India, I don't believe that if someone does not do that, they're doing a bad thing. Not at all. People should realize their inner potential—working anywhere is perfectly fine. There are many ways to give back to your country, and it would be great if we all could contribute in some way. But again, it should be a free choice. There are many problems one can help solve in India and I think there are also very interesting career opportunities available here. I hope more and more people see it in the time to come and return. Not just Indians, but enterprising people from across the globe.

I hope we are able to offer a clean, safe and creative environment for people to stay and work in India. We have many problems, but we also have positives. I think we are getting better as a nation, even if not at a pace that we should. I am confident that we will get there. For me, India is home. I belong here and nothing else matters. Dr Vidushi and I are working to make a difference by giving the gift of sight.

## Practitioner to Entrepreneur

In November 2015, we landed in Delhi and left for Dr Vidushi's home in Noida. We gave ourselves ten days to finalize our plans. Everything was happening too fast. Two days later, my father-in-law invited a few of his friends over for brunch. Most of them were retired officers from the Indian Air Force. When they heard our plans, they were deeply concerned. Their scepticism showed on their faces. 'So, you're going to start your ophthalmic practice in a new city, from scratch, without a plan?' Group Captain (Retd.) B.G. Chitnis asked. Dr Vidushi and I shifted in our seats. I had never felt that uncomfortable in my life. 'You need the five Ps of marketing in place,' Group Capt. Chitnis said. 'Place (hospital), People (team), Patients, Pounds (money), Promotion (Market research).' I reached for my notepad. I noted down his advice while feeling grossly incompetent. But there was no alternative; we had to proceed with our hurriedly drafted plan. Dr Vidushi and I decided to tackle at least a couple of the Ps: pounds and place.

My father-in-law's friends and several others thought that at least we had no shortage of funds. After all, we had just returned after spending several years abroad. What they did not know was that we were early-career fellows earning no more than minimum wage. Almost all our money was spent in rent, travel/accommodation for conferences, instruments, books, utilities and groceries. Still, Dr Vidushi and I had managed to save ₹10 lakhs. We thought this would help us get by for a while but when we reached India, we realized that prices of everything had shot through the roof.

I won't lie, it was scary.

We had to find a way to make things work. So we started looking for non-metro cities that could host our practice. I thought of my ancestral village Mohna and the city closest to it. 'Kota!' I screamed. Dr Vidushi looked up in surprise. 'It's a non-metro, so less expensive, only 70 kms from Mohna, and well-situated in Rajasthan, which means we can treat many patients who complain of eye problems due to the state's harsh sun, dry environment, and widespread sand dust.' I was breathless.

Dr Vidushi smiled and just like that, we had found our place. I made arrangements to visit my younger brother, Dr Rajesh K. Pandey, an Ayurvedic physician, in Jhalawar. From Jhalawar, we planned to go site-hunting in Kota. A Hindi phrase '*khana badosh zindagi*' or nomadic life, came to my mind. In my thirty-seven years, I had lived in nine cities, and here I was, planning to live in my tenth.

A few weeks later, my brother heard of someone who owned an orthopaedic clinic in Kota; Dr M.L. Ahuja had tried to establish his orthopaedic practice for two years but his efforts had not been successful. Hence, he was keen to rent out his newly constructed hospital in one of Kota's new colonies known as Indra Vihar. It was a great location and close to the coaching centres. We fixed a meeting with Dr Ahuja and finalized the agreement.

But this was hardly the end of our battle. The journey to medical entrepreneurship for both of us was no easy task. It's well-known that most doctors end up building their own private practice, but usually, it's a decision that is taken after much deliberation and discussion. Healthcare is a competitive market and healthcare businesses endure many hardships before becoming stable and successful. Any doctor's journey to becoming a successful medical entrepreneur needs more than just an idea and funds to work. When I was working at a university and performing eye surgery, I never thought to check the cost of an operating microscope or equipment such as a phacoemulsifier or LASIK laser machines. For many new doctors, high on idealism and low on finances and family support (in the form of a doctor parent), jumping into private practice is akin to foraying into a jungle—you don't know what to expect. You could be devoured by the wolves or you could find your oasis and prosper. Both of us were jumping headfirst into unknown waters. In an era where people conduct intensive research, consult experts and weigh the pros and cons of everything before deciding to start their own business, we simply made a last-minute emotional decision and embraced the journey as it came.

We had found our hospital building but that wasn't the end of our expenses. We still had to set up the hospital. We were fortunate to get in touch with an expert operation theater (OT) technician. With his help, we were able to initiate the setup of an OT. But we needed equipment. We decided to meet up with Mariappan Pillai from Appasamy Associates (Chennai), who were leading manufacturers and distributors of ophthalmic equipment. We told Mr Pillai about our plan to start our practice in Kota and asked him to provide us with the necessary equipment. He assured us that he would make an ophthalmic chair unit, slit lamp biomicroscopy, auto refractometer, lensometer, direct and indirect ophthalmoscopes available to us. But the total cost of those would come up to about ₹10 lakhs. We approached a bank for a loan but the bank manager asked us for two years of tax returns filed in India, as well as assets in our name that we could mortgage. We had neither and so the bank refused us the loan. We returned to Appasamy and requested him if he could defer the payment for one year, which he told us he would have to check with their head office. A ringing silence followed for days, till one day, when Mr Pillai called and told us that our request had been approved. Dr Vidushi and I rejoiced that we could start seeing patients.

## Setting up the Hospital

We chose to rent Dr Ahuja's building not only because we could have our hospital on the ground floor, but also because we could use the floor above as our residence. The ground floor consisted of a reception area, two OPD consultation chambers, a ward with four beds, one minor operation theatre, one major operation theatre with one operating table, an Emergency Room, a spectacle shop and a pharmacy. Now that we had a few machines, the ground floor had started looking like a hospital.

But this was the bare minimum. We desperately needed a phacoemulsification system to perform suture-less cataract surgery. We could not afford it but we decided to take a risk and spend our remaining savings on this machine. We cut back on expenditure in other ways. We hired only three employees—Hemraj Meghwanshi, our OT technician, an OPD assistant and a receptionist. We maintained a small team and had insufficient support staff. This meant that we performed a majority of the tasks ourselves. We did not hire an optometrist, and Dr Vidushi would test the power of lenses herself. She would also calculate the lens power for cataract surgery cases, and assist in the operating room. But there was a deeper thought behind ensuring that we did all the small tasks in the hospital. We had just returned from Australia but we did not want our patients to feel that we were too highbrow and they could not connect with us. We made it a point to be friendly and approachable to all our patients. We had decided to name our practice SuVi (shortened form of Suresh and Vidushi) Eye Hospital.

A few patients came in with cataracts and I would step in to perform their cataract surgery. I was used to performing the surgery with a high-end operating microscope that would have cost us ₹60 lakhs. But there was no way we could afford it. So we purchased an imported, lower-end Carl Zeiss, Germany operating microscope instead. It took me a few days to get used to the new AMO compact, USA phaco machine and a new operating microscope. In Australia, most of the investigation was done by ophthalmic assistants. Here, Dr Vidushi would calculate the power of the lens and record the Keratometry (K) Reading herself, using a manual keratometer. We would put the dilating eye drop in the eyes of patients ourselves and each patient would undergo a complete retina examination. We would check if the pupils were dilated and would then explain the disease to the patient and their attendant in detail.

We decided that even if we didn't have a sound financial plan, we would use the best clinical practices possible to keep our patients satisfied. We were now realistic in our quest and had mentally prepared ourselves for the challenges that would be coming our way.

But the odds were stacked against us since we had started off without a plan, or an alternate plan. Being experts in clinical and surgical work, with years of experience and international exposure, we were unaware of the business side of medical practice. But now we had rolled the dice, all we could do now was wait for patients to show up.

# 12

# Leaping Over Roadblocks

## Creating a Brand

*'Imagination is everything. It is the preview of life's coming attractions.'*
—Albert Einstein

## Healing Touch in the New Year

It was early morning on 1 January 2007 when our night staff received a phone call from an elderly patient. The caller said that his wife was experiencing severe pain in both eyes. The pain was unbearable and did not subside even after taking painkillers. His wife had started crying with pain in the middle of the night and he was feeling helpless. He had consulted an eye doctor on the previous day, who had not been able to find the precise cause of her pain. The doctor told them it could be a psychosomatic or neurological pain, and so had asked them to consult a neurologist and psychiatrist. Their family lived abroad and the elderly couple lived all alone. At 3 A.M., my staff member woke me up. I was at Sudha Hospital, Kota, at the time. A few hours back, Dr Vidushi had undergone an emergency caesarean section and our daughter Ishita was born in December 2006. I came

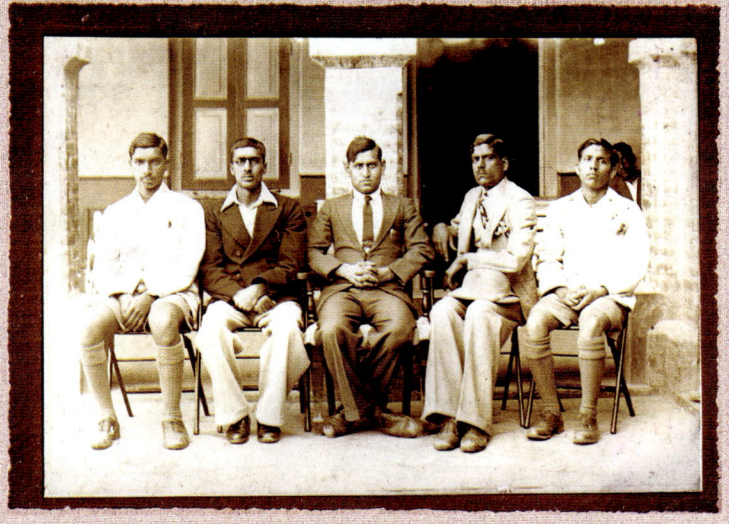

**K. J. F. EYE HOSPITAL**
BHIWANI
1937

**SURGEONS & POST GRADUATES**
Left to Right :- 1. K.N. Dwivedi, 2. Dr. H. R. Dewan, 3. Dr. P. D. Giridhar
V.B.S   L.M.P.(C.P.)   Ophth. Surgeon I/C.
4. Dr. S. C. Misra, 5. Dr. Kamta Prasad Pandey

Figure 1. My dadaji, freedom fighter and renowned eye surgeon Dr Kamta Prasad Pandey with Dr P.D. Giridhar (Chief Eye Surgeon) and other eye surgeons at Kishan Lal Jalan Eye Hospital, Bhiwani (Haryana, India), 1937.

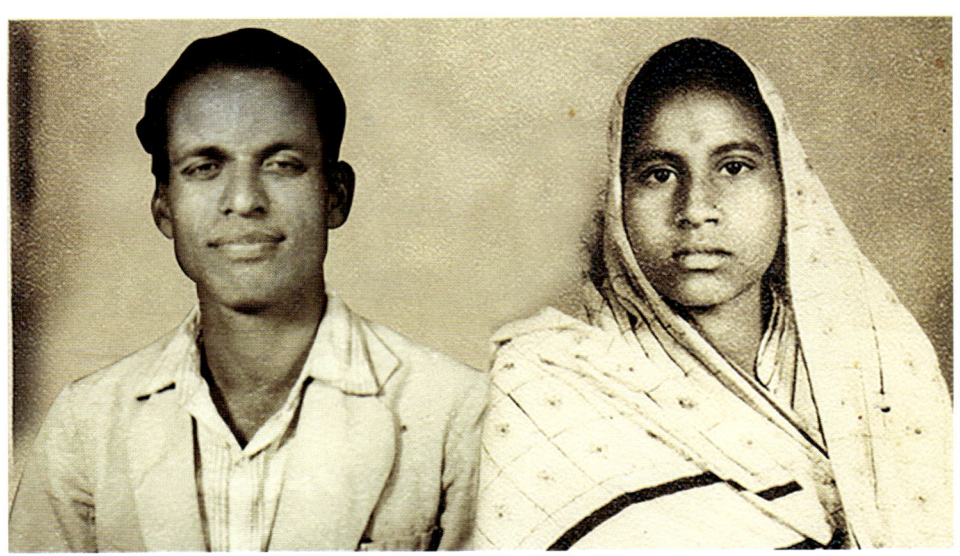

Figure 2. My parents, Late Shri Kameshwar Prasad Pandey and Late Smt. Maya Devi Pandey, 1973.

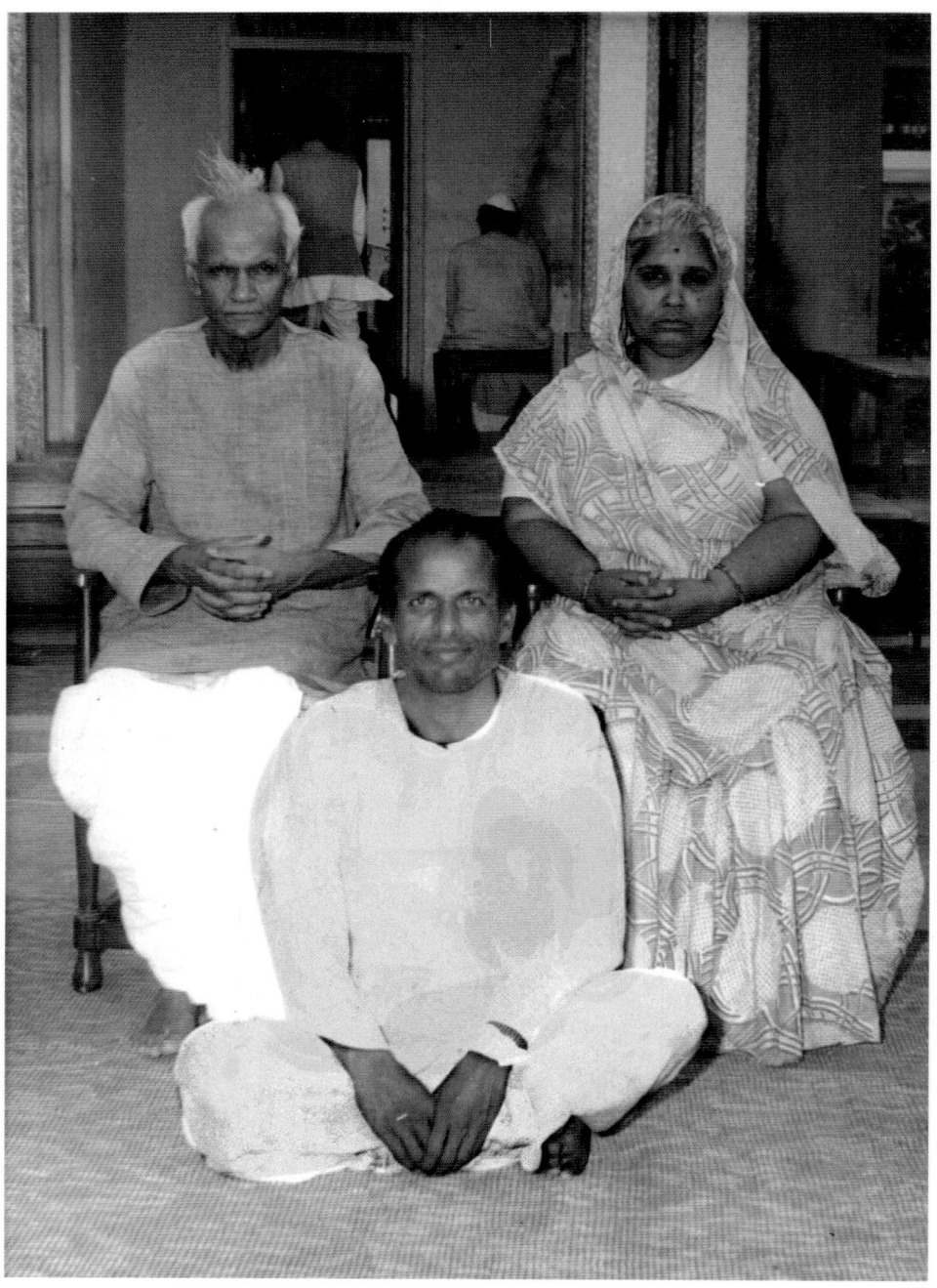

Figure 3. My father receiving the blessings of respected Gurudev Acharya Shri Ram Sharma and revered Mataji Smt. Bhagwati Devi Sharma during the Gayatri Sadhna Camp at Gayatri Tapobhoomi, Mathura, 1968.

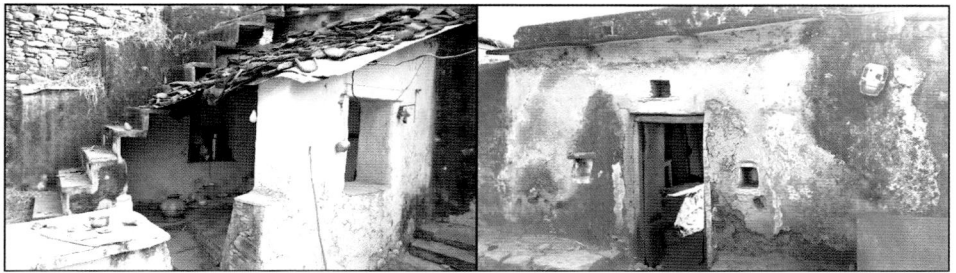

Figure 4. Our old house situated in Mohna village, where I resided from 1968 to 1982.

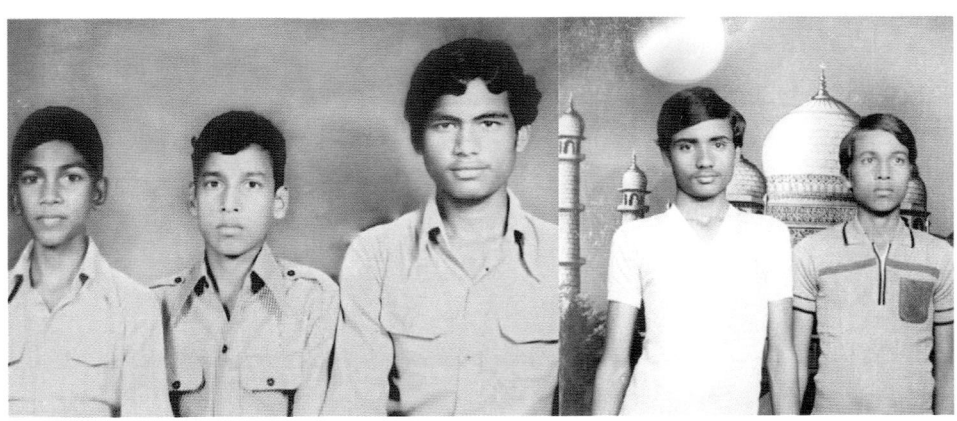

Figure 5. Some of my classmates and close friends from Rawatbhata School, 1983. From left to right: Dr Dinesh Birla (Professor, Rajasthan Technical University, Kota), me and Dhirendra Kumar Jain (Professor, Polytechnic College, Kota). In the adjoining picture, Shri Rameshwar Prasad Gupta (State Bank of India) and me.

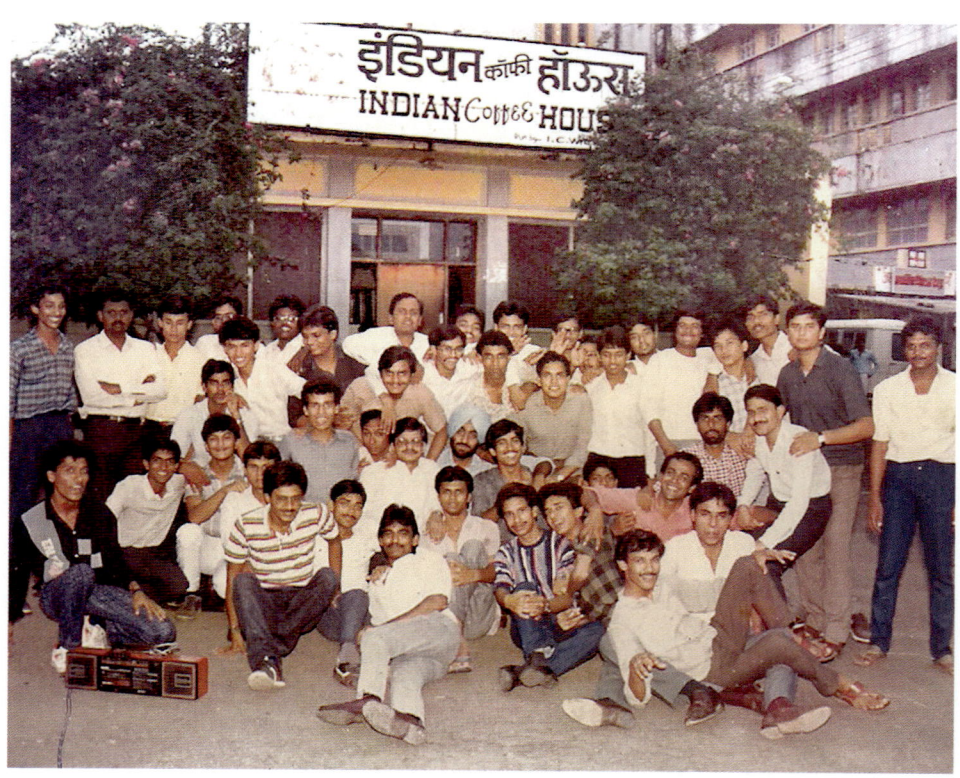

Figure 6. With our hostel seniors in front of the Indian Coffee House, Medical College, Jabalpur campus, November 1986.

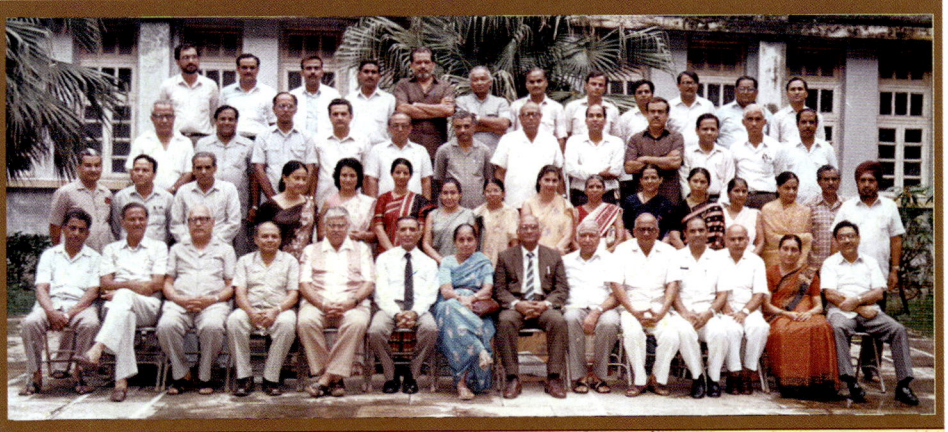

FAREWELL TO
# Dr. B.B.L. Mathur, Dean, Govt. Medical College, Jabalpur
ON HIS RETIREMENT ON 31-5-1988

Sitting on chairs L to R—S/Shri V.S.C Rao. B.M. Arora. K.P Chansoriya. R.K Gupta K.R. Munjal. B.B.b. Mathur, Mrs S Deshpande, S.N. Shrivastave, Dr. T.M. Garg, D.K. Gupta, H.D. Siddiqui J.P. Kapoor. Mrs. I Datt K K. Kaul.

Standing 1st row L to R—J.K. Tandon, M.P. Gupta G.P. Vyas, Miss. B. Mukherjee. Mrs. S Munjal. Miss. Maya Chansoriya. Miss. A. Kaur Smt. S. Khare, Mrs K. Hasceja, Mrs. N. Bhatnagar, Dr. A Leie, Mrs. A Dixit, Mrs. R Srivastava Miss H. Subedar, M.A. Hafeez. Surinder Singh.

Standing 2nd row L to R—G.S. Mehtab, B.K. Jain. S.K. Verma B.P. Singh. J.K Sharma D,K. Shrivastava, S.b. Mukherjee S. Thora. A.K. Mukherjee, M. Bhatnagar, S.M. Tejwani, A.N. Joshi.

Standing 3rd row L to R—Arun Sharma. V.K. Mehta, A.K. Dubey. B.P. Tikria, A.S. Rathore R C. Agarwal. L.P. Ahirwar. V.K. Raina. D.K Sakaliey, S.K. Shrivastava, T. Ghosh. K,D,Baghel.

[Sharma Colour Lab,

Figure 7. Group photograph on the occasion of the retirement of Professor B.B.L. Mathur (Dean and Head of the Department of Physiology) with our esteemed faculty from various departments of Medical College, Jabalpur, 1988.

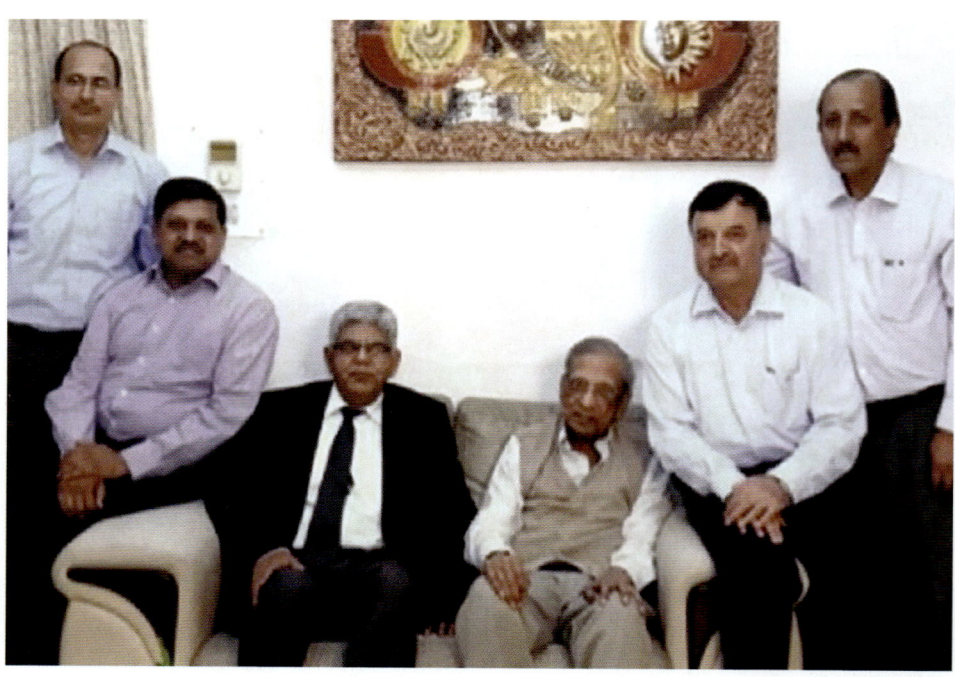

Figure 8. The five heads of the ophthalmology department, PGIMER, Chandigarh in one picture. From left to right: Dr S.S. Pandav, Dr Sandeep Jain, Dr Amod Gupta, Dr Inder Sen Jain, Dr Mangat Ram Dogra, and Dr Jagat Ram.

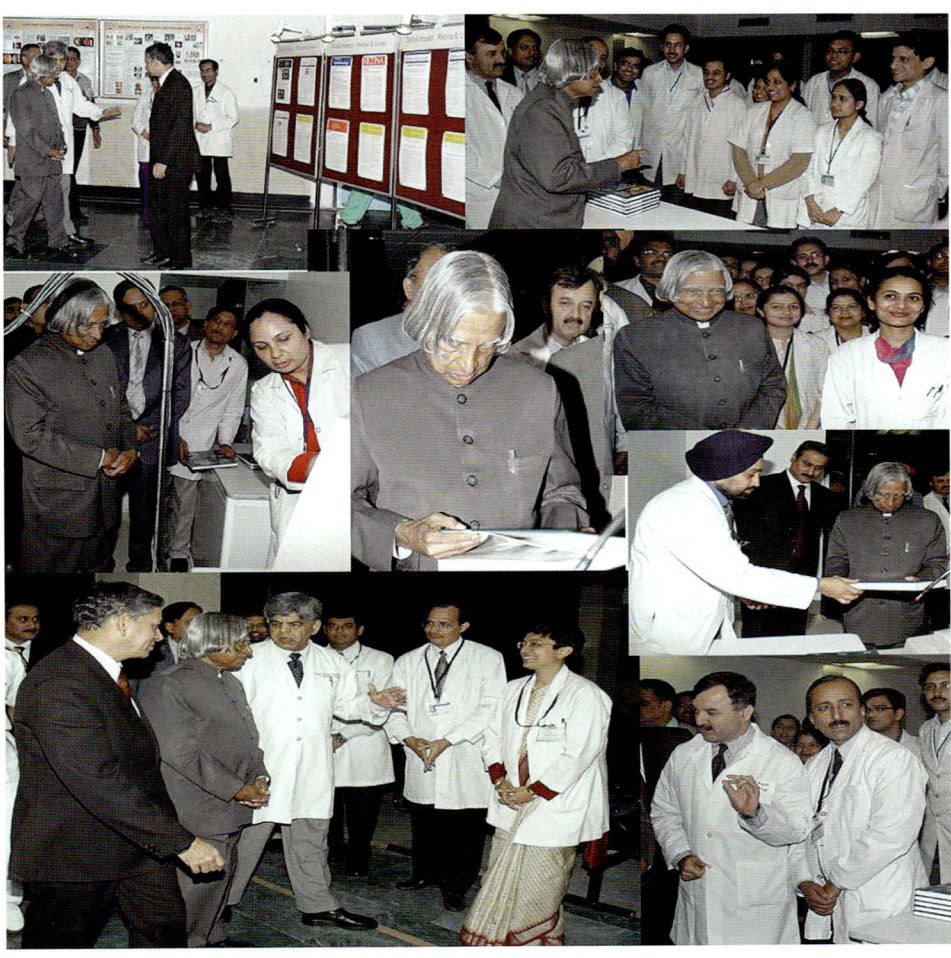

Figure 9. Visit of Bharat Ratna Dr A.P.J. Abdul Kalam at Advanced Eye Centre, PGIMER Chandigarh on 8 March 2007. Dr Amod Gupta explained to him the clinical and research work done by the faculty members of the AEC.

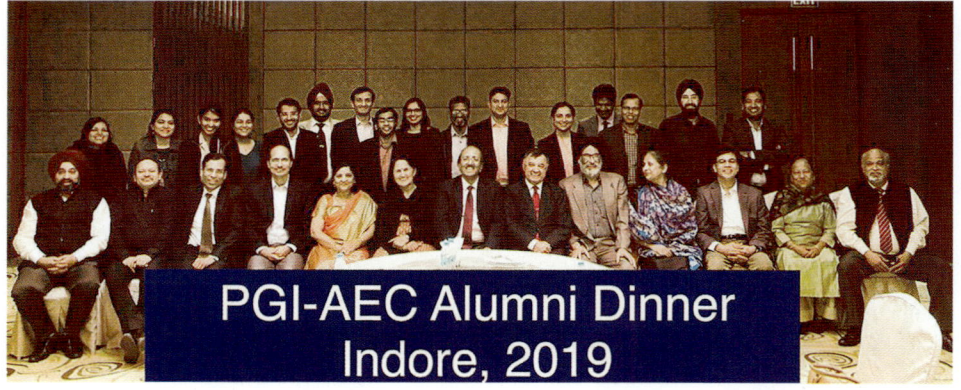

Figure 10. The PGIMER, Chandigarh, Advanced Eye Centre (AEC) Alumni dinner was held during the All India Ophthalmology Conference, Indore. Pictured here are my respected teachers at AEC, Dr Jagat Ram, Dr M.R. Dogra, Dr S.S. Pandav and Dr Usha Singh, seniors and classmates.

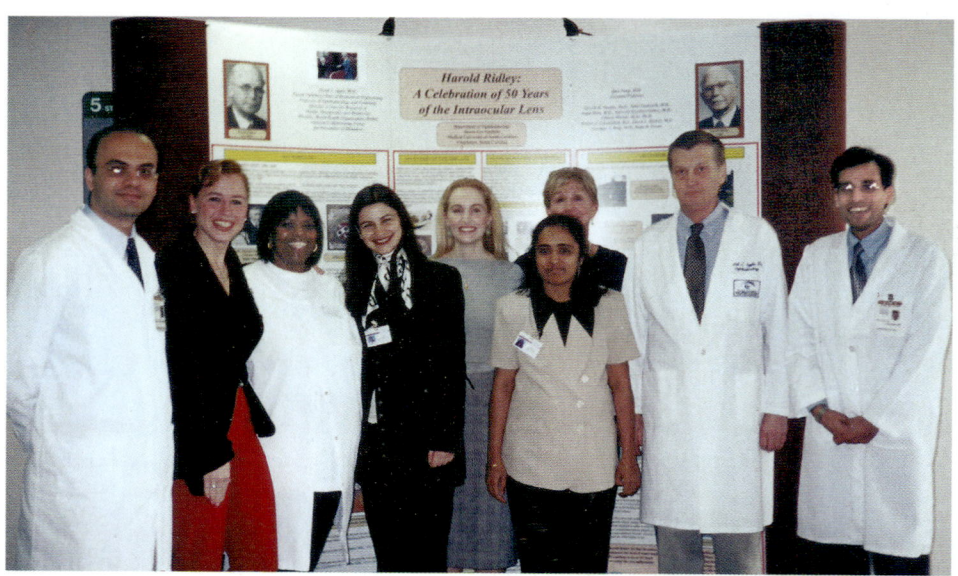

Figure 11. 'The Apple Korps'. From right to left: Dr Suresh K. Pandey (India), Professor David J. Apple, Dr Rupal H. Trivedi (India), Dr Liliana Werner (Brazil), Dr Andrea M. Izakova (Czechoslovakia) and Dr Tamer A. Mackey (Egypt).

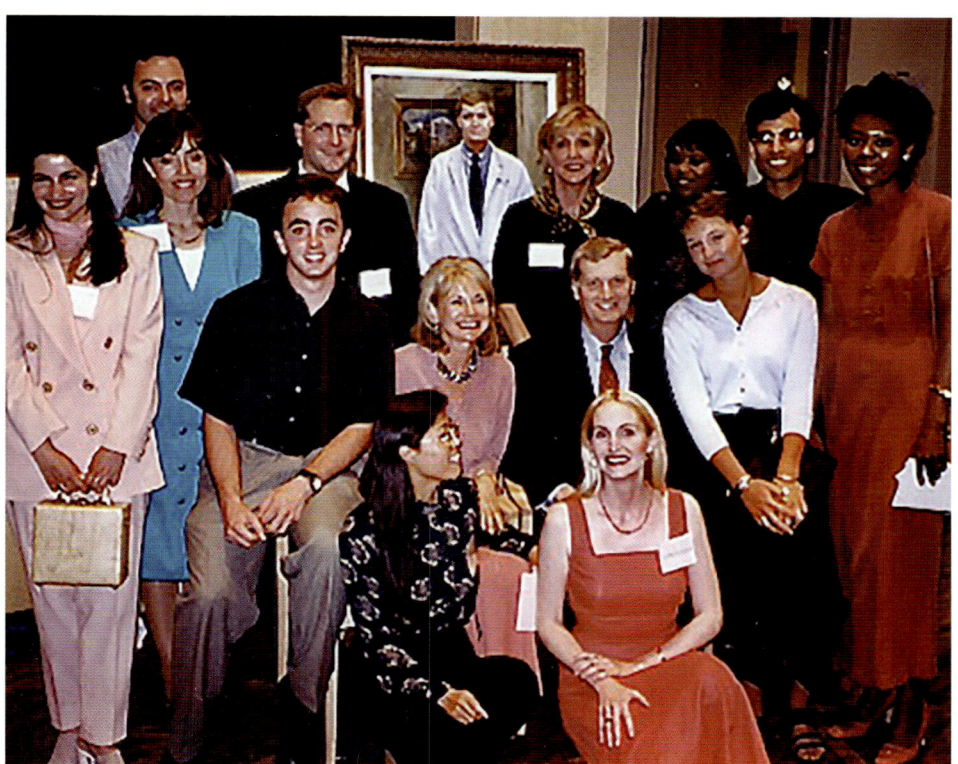

Figure 12. Dr David J. Apple and his wife, Anne Apple with the Apple Korps. Seen in the photo are (Left to right, first row, sitting) Dr Qun Peng and Daphne Hoddinott. (Left to right, second row, sitting) Beau Evans, Ann Apple, Dr David J. Apple, Lucia McLendon. (Left to right, third row, standing) Dr Liliana Werner, Dr Marcela Escobar-Gomez, Dr Gerd Auffarth, Maddie Manuel, Dr Stella M. Arthur. (Left to right, last row, standing) Dr Roberto Bianchi, Joyce Edmonds and me.

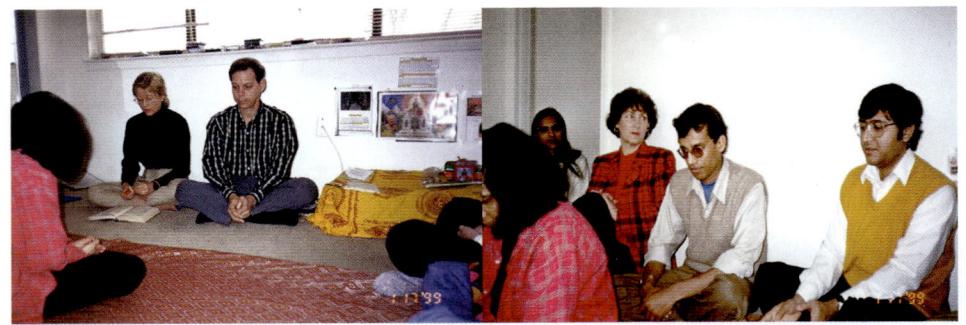

Figure 13. During one of the two-hour satsangs we organized every Sunday morning from 10 AM–12 PM. I would cook pooris and pakoras on these occasions.

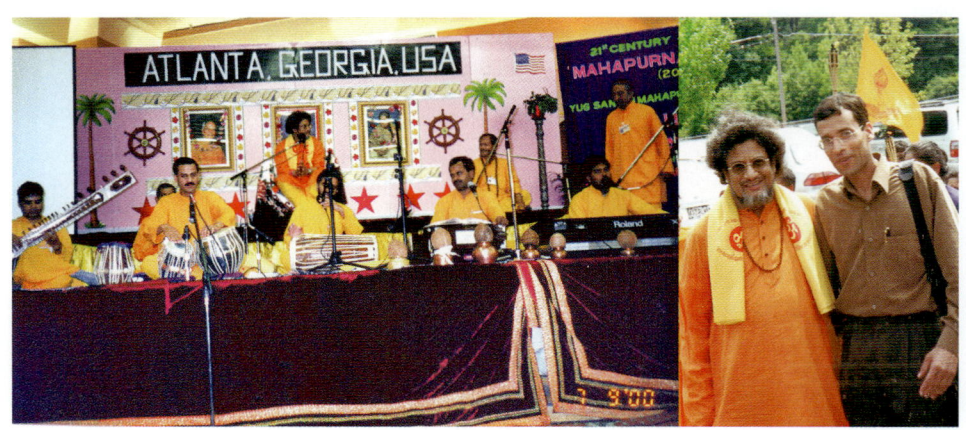

Figure 14. I participated in the Gayatri Ashvamedh Yagya in Atlanta, USA, on 9 July 2000. I got the opportunity to meet Dr Pranav Pandya, Head of Shantikunj, Haridwar, and All World Gayatri Parivar.

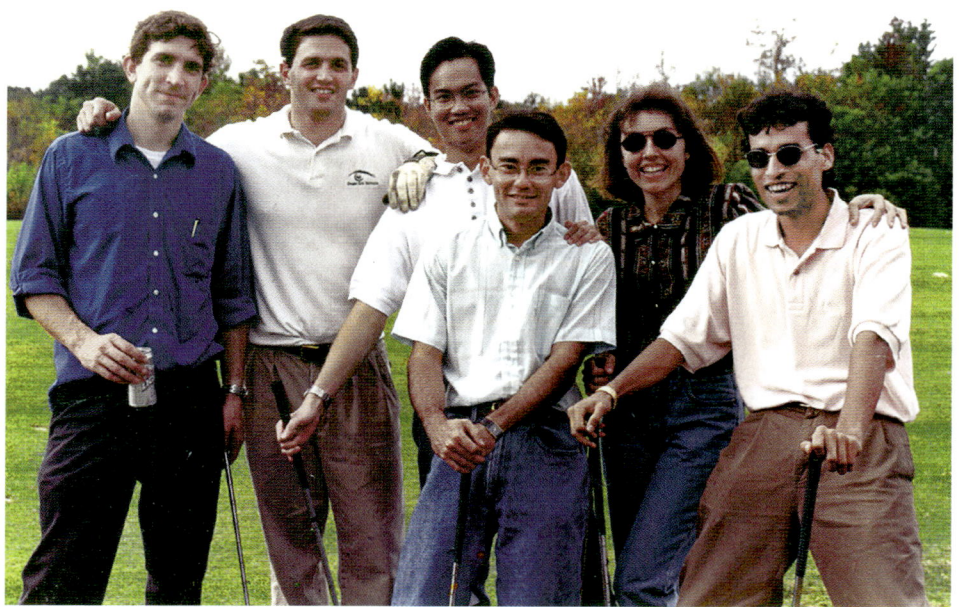

Figure 15. My colleagues and I used to play football or golf on Sundays in line with our motto of 'Work Hard, Play Hard'.

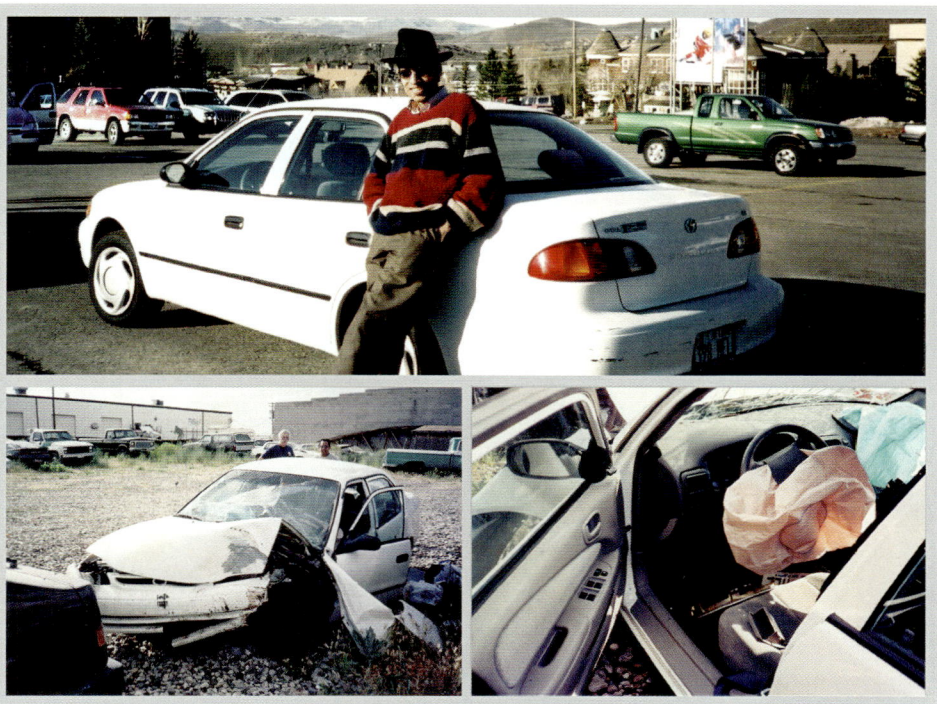

Figure 16. My Toyota Corolla and its condition after my near-fatal car accident on 8 September 2002, in Salt Lake City, USA. The incident solidified in my mind the importance of safe driving, wearing seatbelts and getting enough sleep before driving.

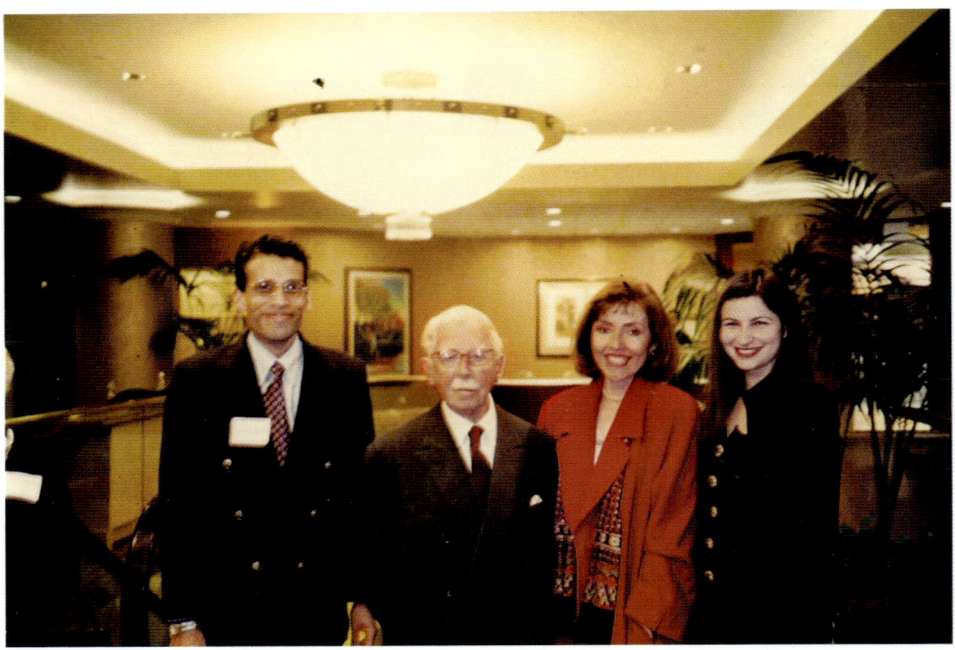

Figure 17. Me with Sir Harold Ridley, the inventor of the intraocular lens. Left to right: me, Sir Harold Ridley, Dr Marcella Escobar-Gomez and Dr Liliana Werner, during the American Society of Cataract and Refractive Surgery (ASCRS) conference in Seattle, USA, April 1999.

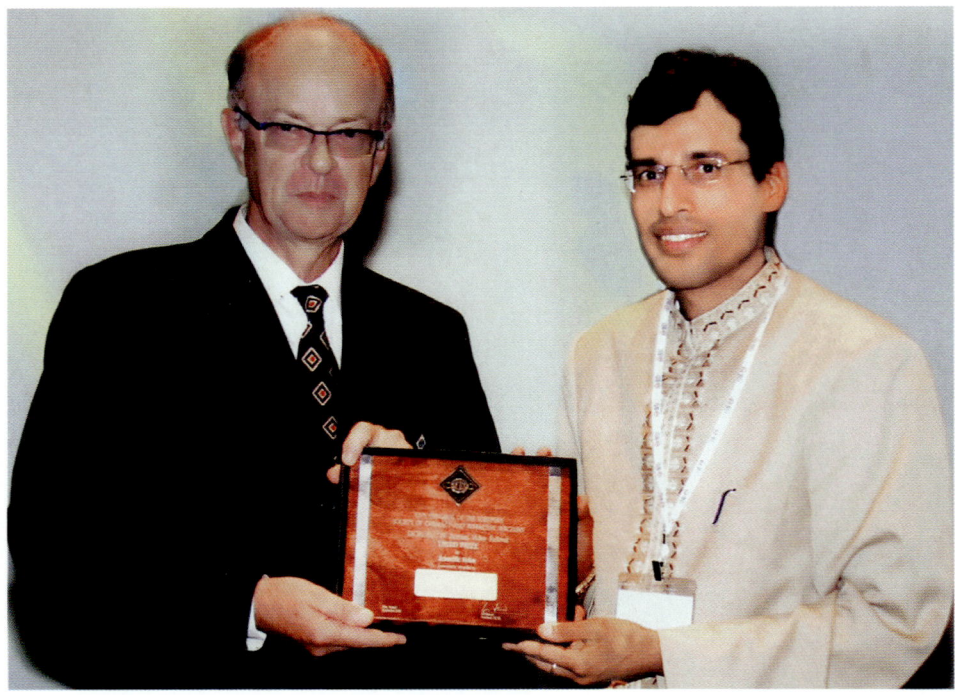

Figure 18. Receiving the ESCRS Film Festival award at the European Society of Cataract and Refractive Surgery (ESCRS) Conference in Vienna, Austria, September 1999.

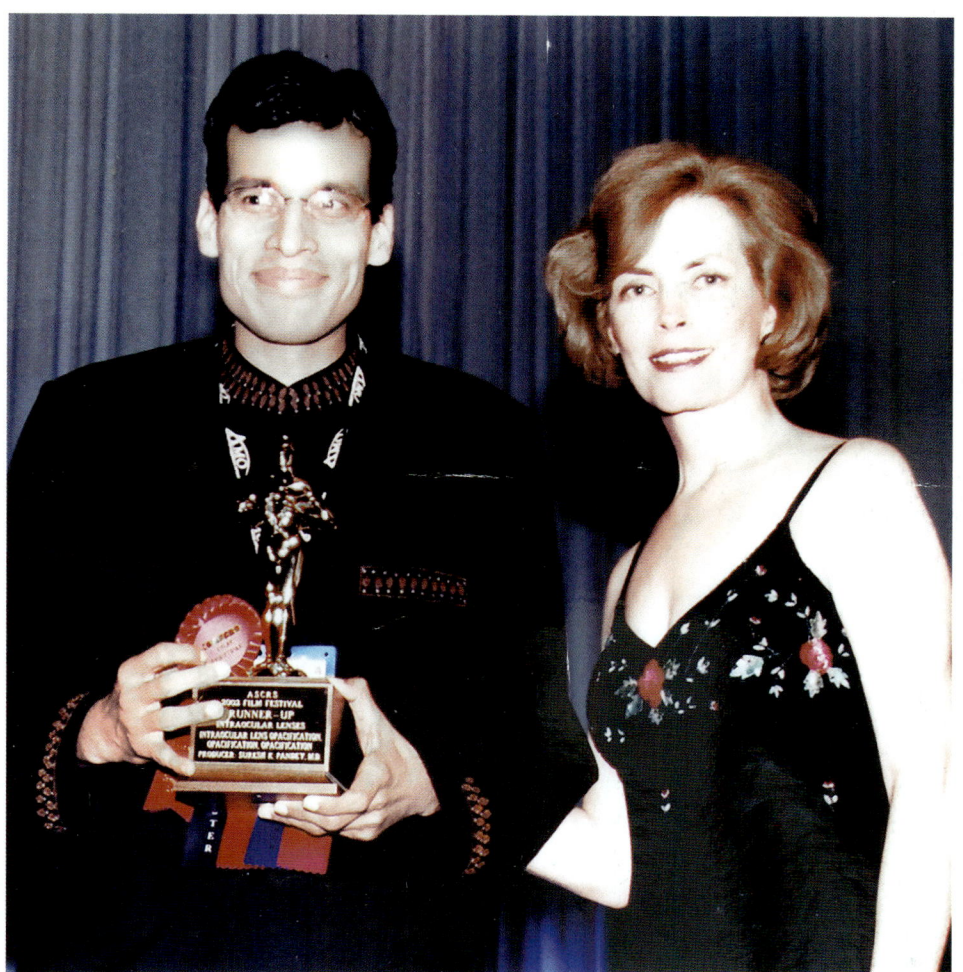

Figure 19. Receiving an American Society of Cataract and Refractive Surgery film festival award at the ASCRS Conference in San Diego, USA, May 2001.

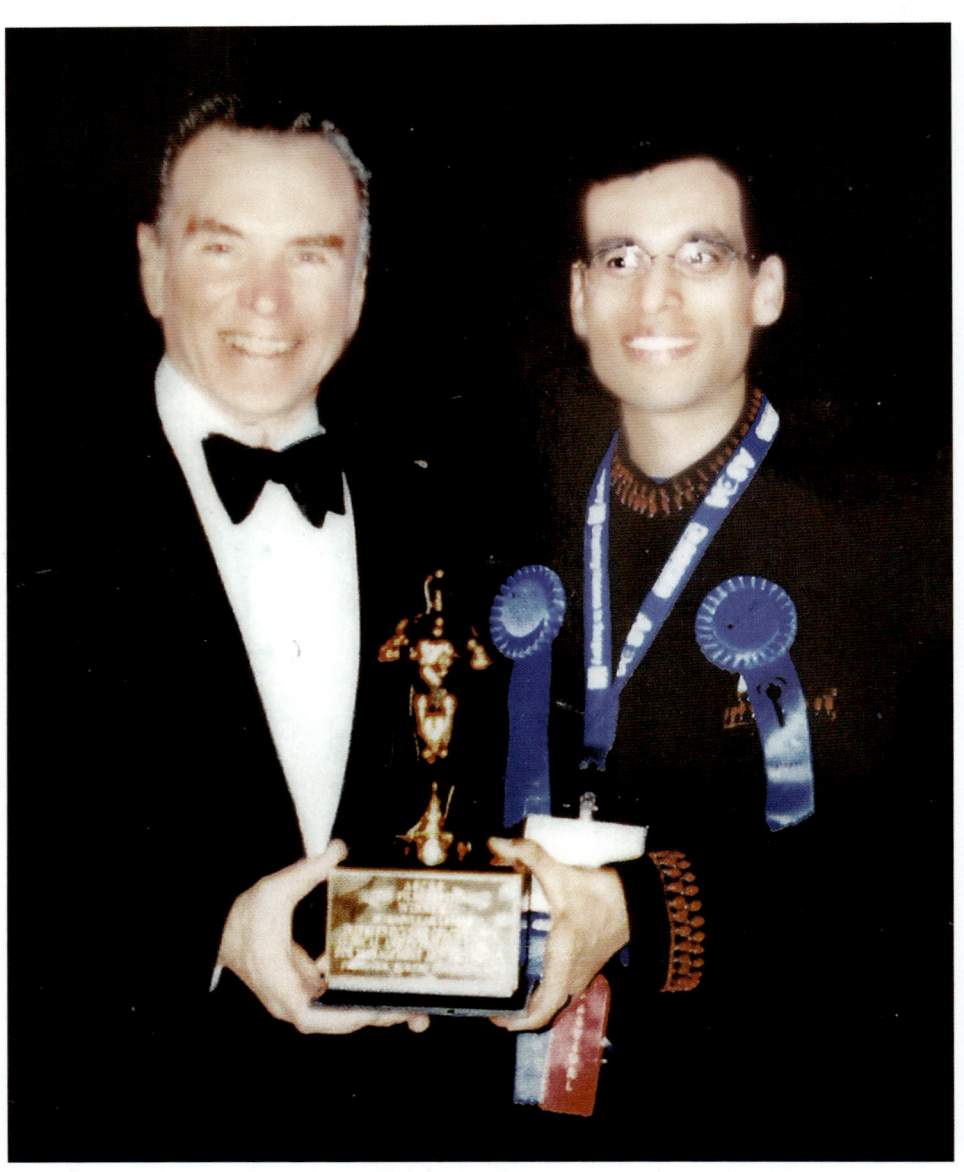

Figure 20. Receiving the Best Video Award at the ASCRS Conference in Boston, USA, May 2000.

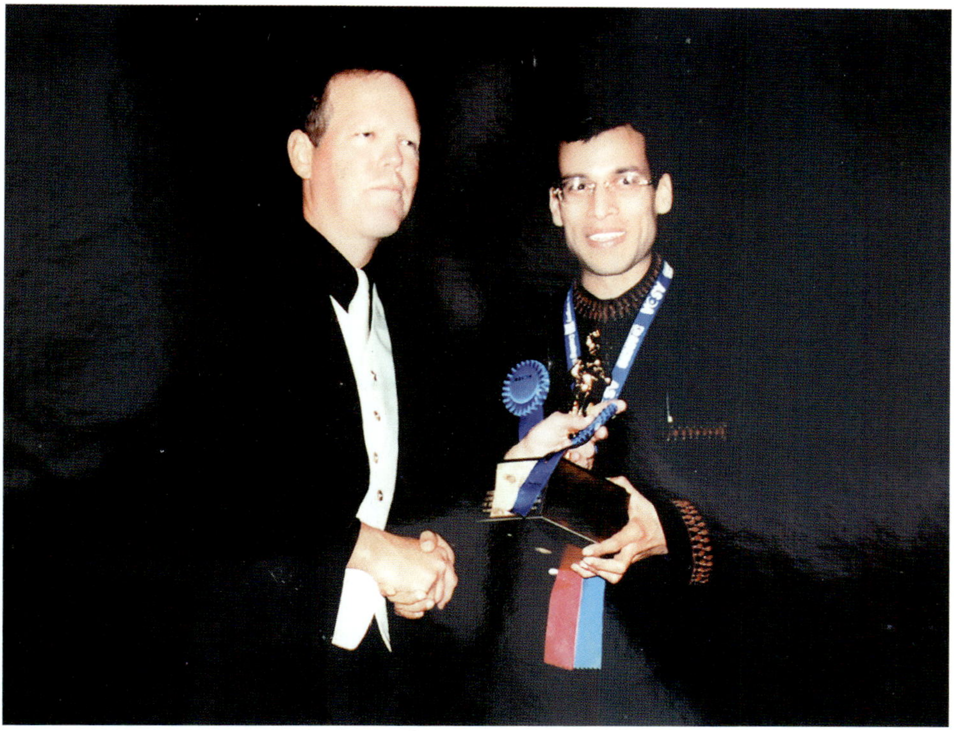

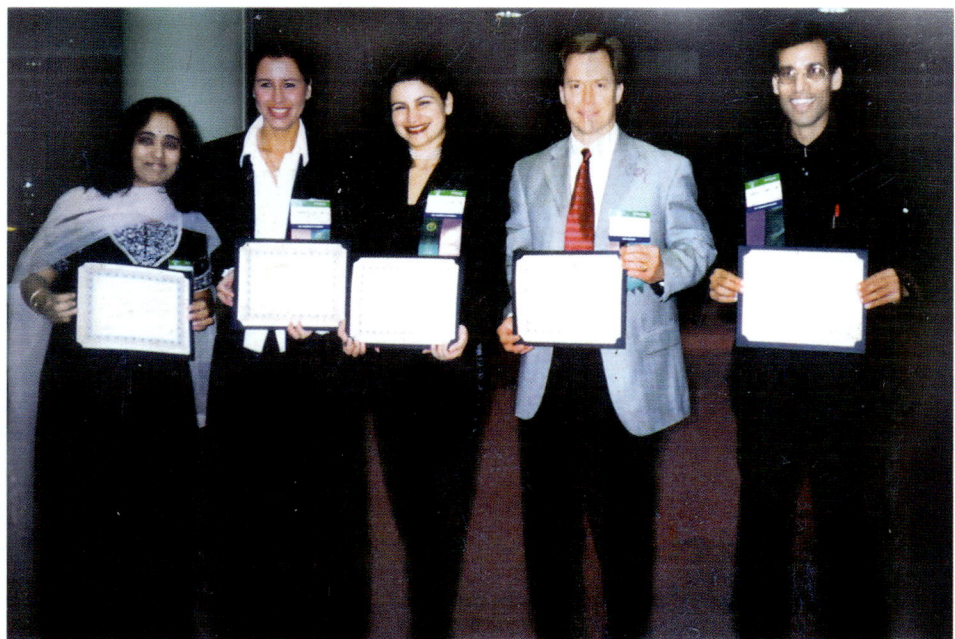

Figure 21. Receiving the Best Video Award during the ASCRS Conference in Philadelphia, USA, June 2002.

Figure 22. Me and my co-authors received the Best of Show Video Award at the Annual Conference of the American Academy of Ophthalmology in Orlando, Florida, USA, October 2002.

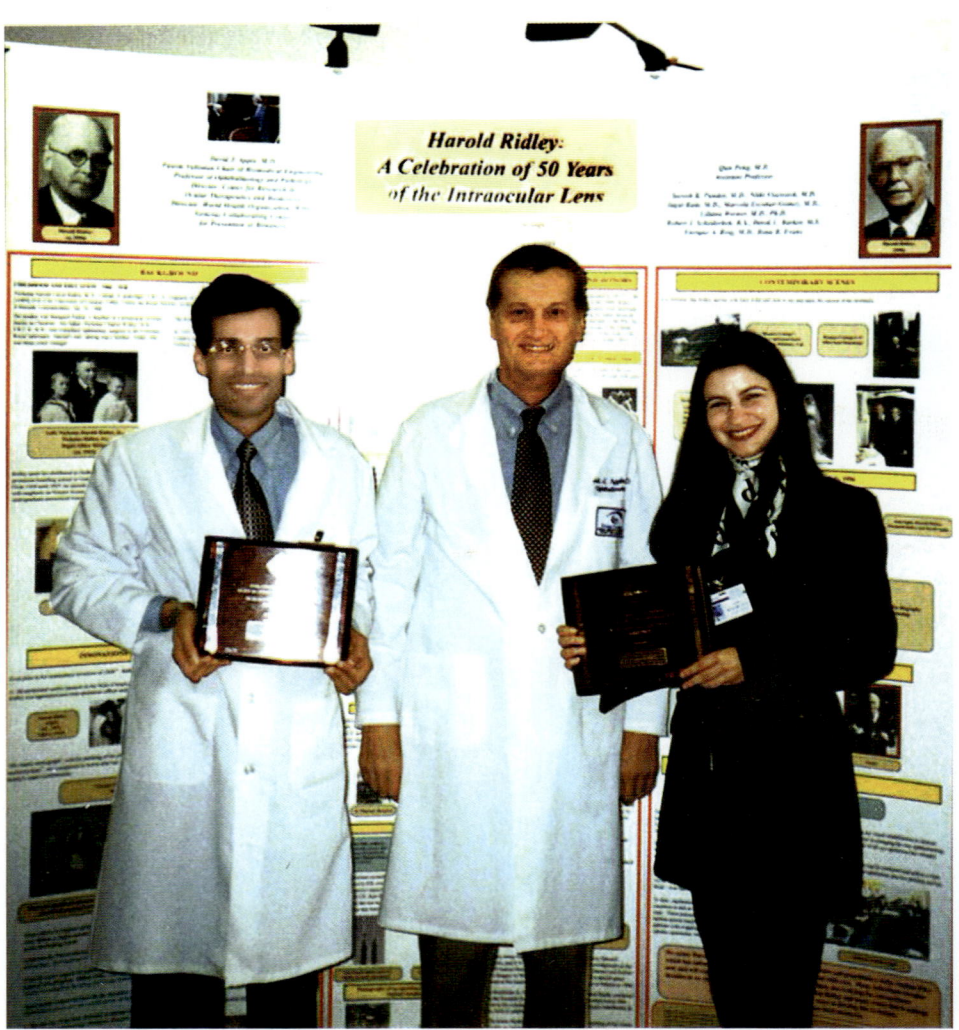

Figure 23. Me, Professor David J. Apple and Dr Liliana Werner at Storm Eye Institute, MUSC campus after receiving the Video Award during the European Society of Cataract and Refractive Surgeons (ESCRS) Conference in Brussels, Belgium, September 2000.

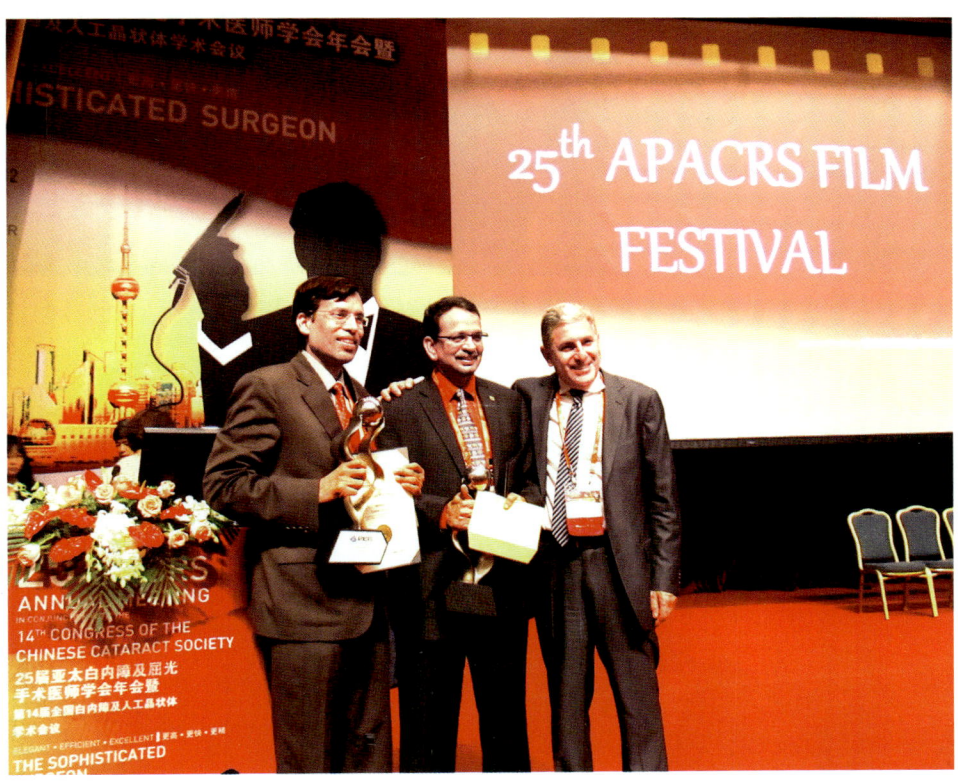

Figure 24. I received the Video Award from Dr Graham Barrett during the Asia Pacific Association of Cataract and Refractive Surgeons (APACRS) Conference in Shanghai, China, May–June 2012.

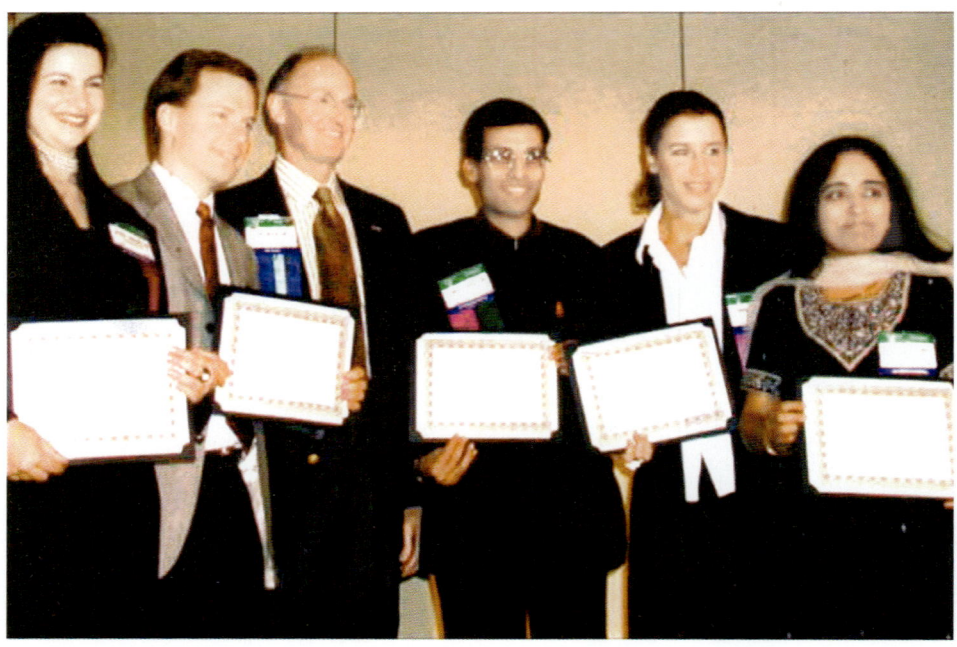

Figure 25. My co-authors and I received the Best of Show Award at the Annual Conference of the American Academy of Ophthalmology in New Orleans, USA, November 2001.

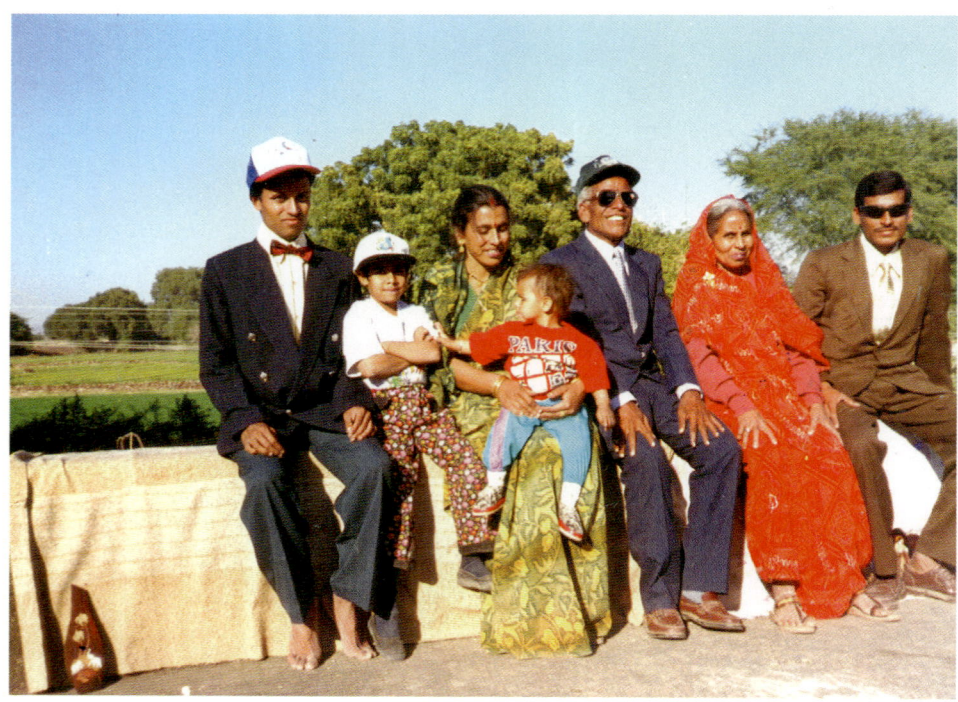

Figure 26. A picture of my family members I clicked during my visit to India, 2000. From left to right: Dr Dinesh K. Pandey, Dr Shivangi Dwivedi, Smt. Usha Pandey, Dr Umang Dwivedi, Shri Kameshwar Prasad Pandey, Smt. Maya Pandey and Dr Rajesh K. Pandey.

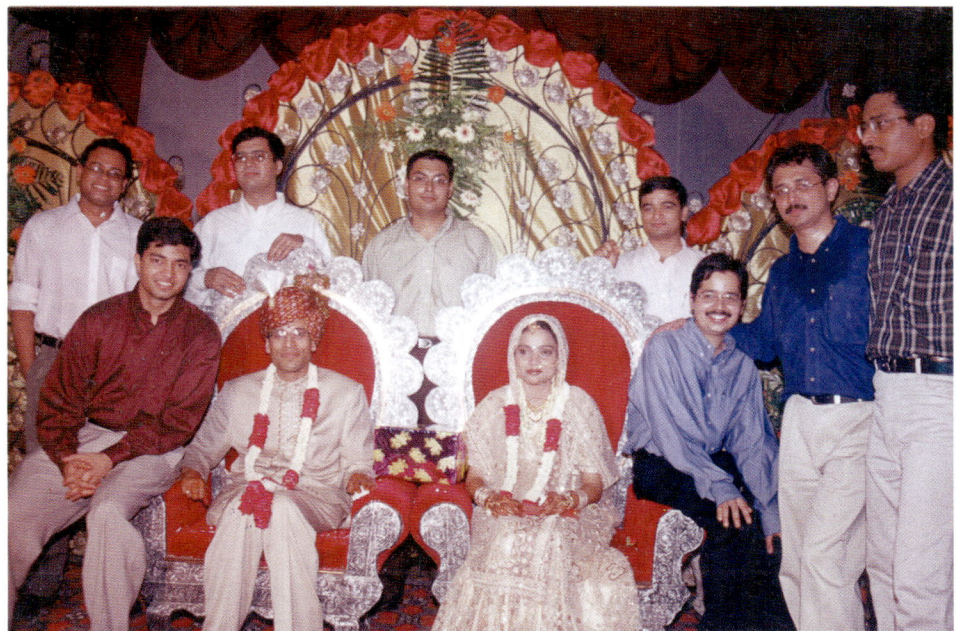

Figure 27. From Dr Vidushi and my wedding in June 2002 at Community Centre, Sector 53, Noida. Also pictured here are Dr Vidushi's colleagues, Dr Prashant Bharatiya, Dr Gunjan Prakash and Dr Amol Kulkarni.

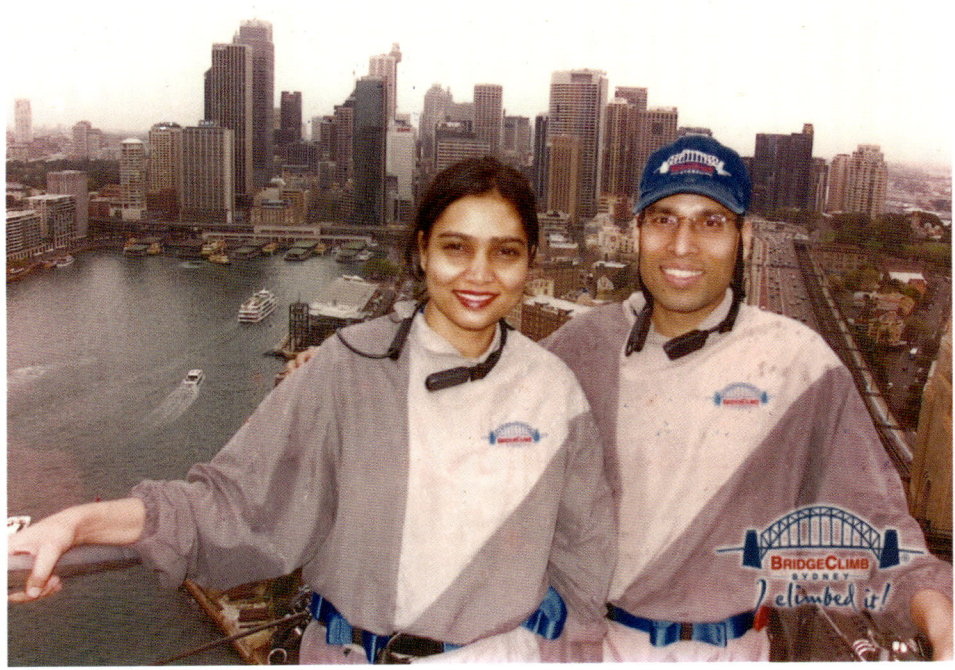

Figure 28. Dr Vidushi and I on one of our weekend expeditions at the Sydney Harbour bridge, Sydney, Australia.

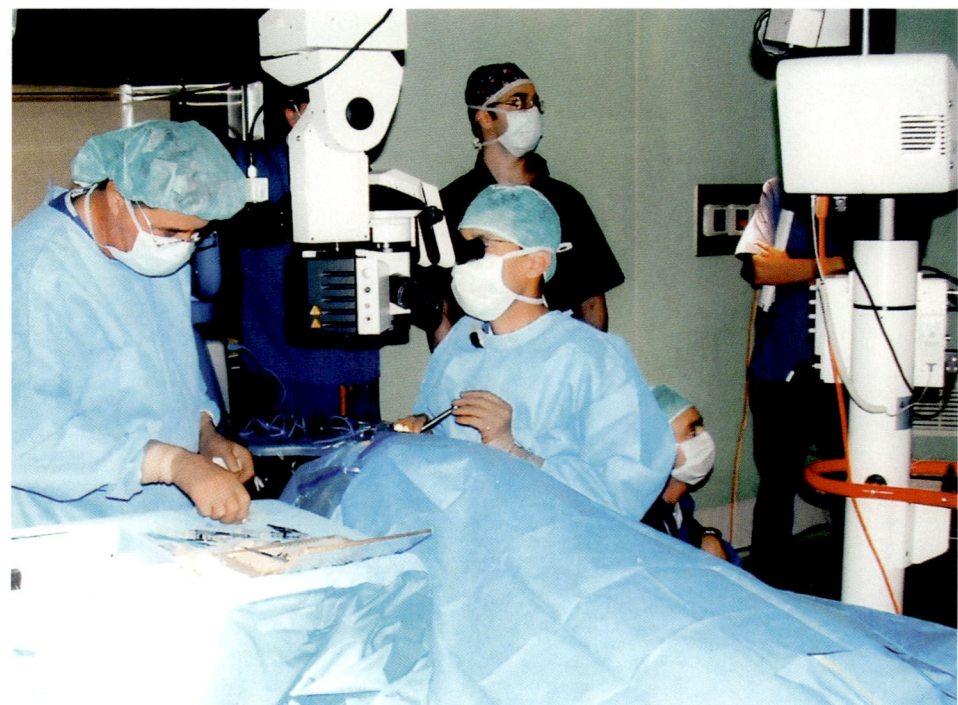

Figure 29. '*Guarda la luce*' ('Look into the light'), I told my patient during my first international live surgery in Milan, Italy on 28 October 2005. The live surgery event was organized at the Centro Ambrosiano di Microchirurgia Oculare (or CAMO, now known as the clinic Centro Ambrosiano Oftalmico)—one of the most famous eye institutes in Milan—by Dr Lucio Buratto.

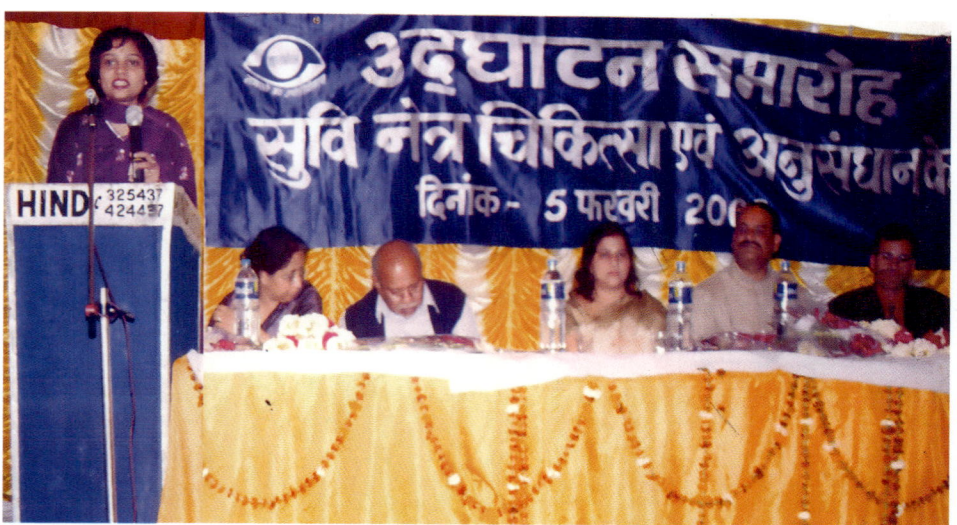

Figure 30. The inauguration of SuVi Eye Hospital, Kota, 5 February 2006. Left to right: Dr Vidushi Sharma (podium), Smt. Ghosh, Professor Supriyo Ghosh (Chief of Dr Rajendra Prasad Centre for Ophthalmic Sciences, All India Institute of Medical Sciences [AIIMS], New Delhi), Dr Amita Birla, Shri Om Birla (current Lok Sabha Speaker) and me.

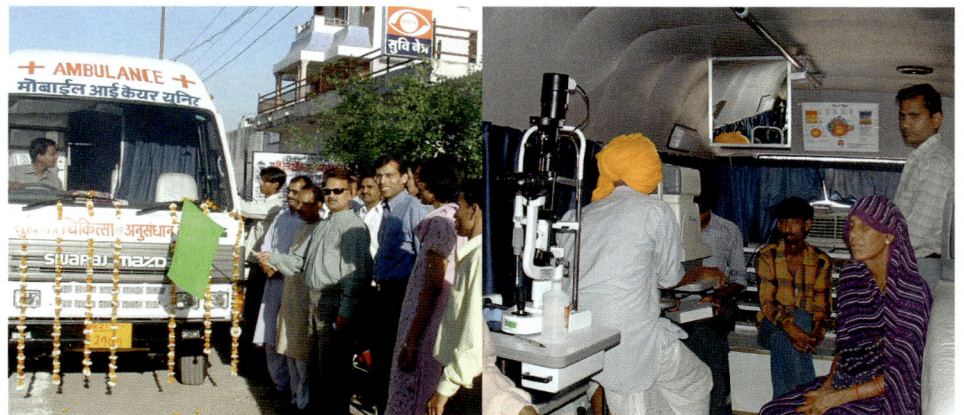

Figure 31. The Mobile Eye Care Unit of SuVi Eye Hospital being flagged off by the then District Collector Shri Niranjan Arya, wearing sunglasses here, in March 2006.

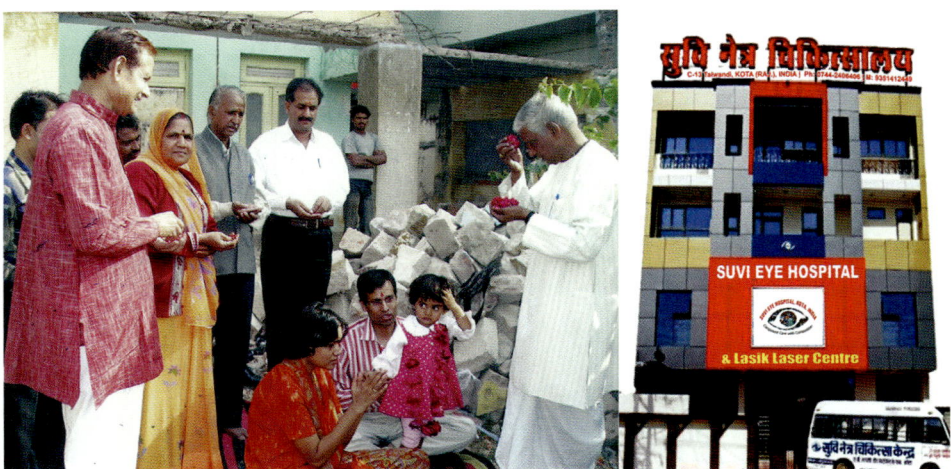

Figure 32. Left: Bhoomi poojan before the construction of the new building of SuVi Eye Hospital, Kota began. Right: The completed hospital building.

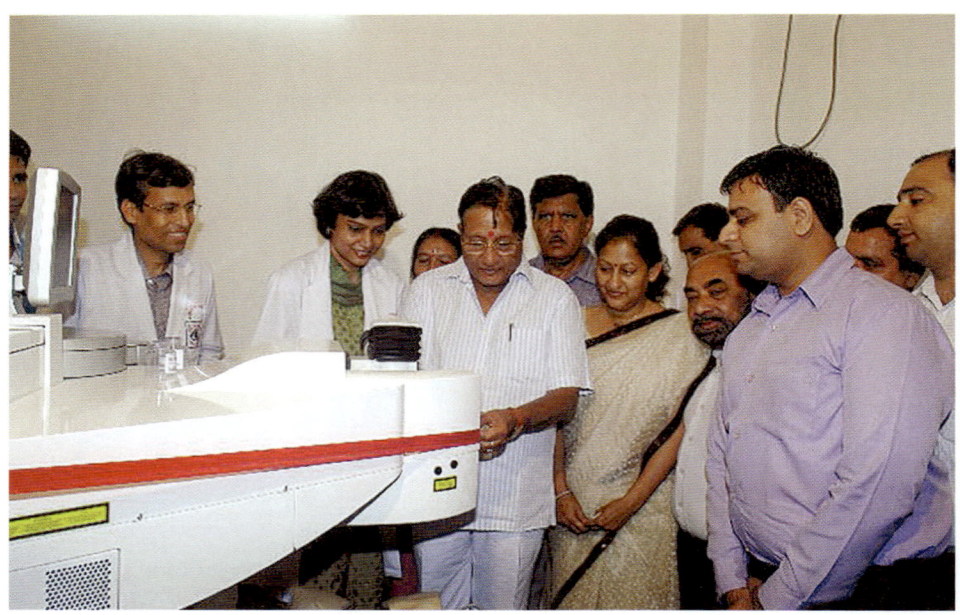

Figure 33. Inauguration of the NASA-certified Visx LASIK laser refractive surgery machine at SuVi Eye Hospital, Kota,15 August 2011 by the Urban Development and Housing Minister of Rajasthan, Shri Shanti Kumar Dhariwal. Left to Right: me, Dr Vidushi Sharma, Shri Shanti Kumar Dhariwal (UDH Minister), Shri Ravindra Tyagi (UIT Chairman), Dr Ratna Jain (Mayor, Kota City), Shri Arun Bhargava, Shri Chandraveer Singh Chauhan (Johnson & Johnson Vision), Shri Rajesh Pandit (Johnson & Johnson Vision).

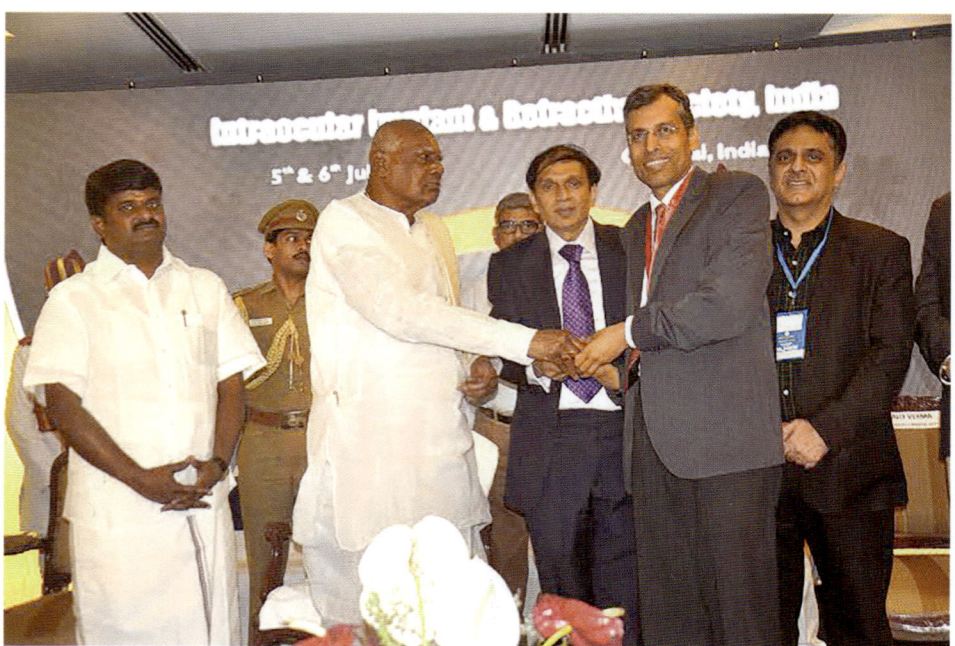

Figure 34. I received a gold medal for doing excellent work in the field of cataract-IOL surgery from the Governor and Health Minister of Tamil Nadu during the Intraocular Implant and Refractive Society, India (IIRSI) Conference in Chennai, India, July 2014.

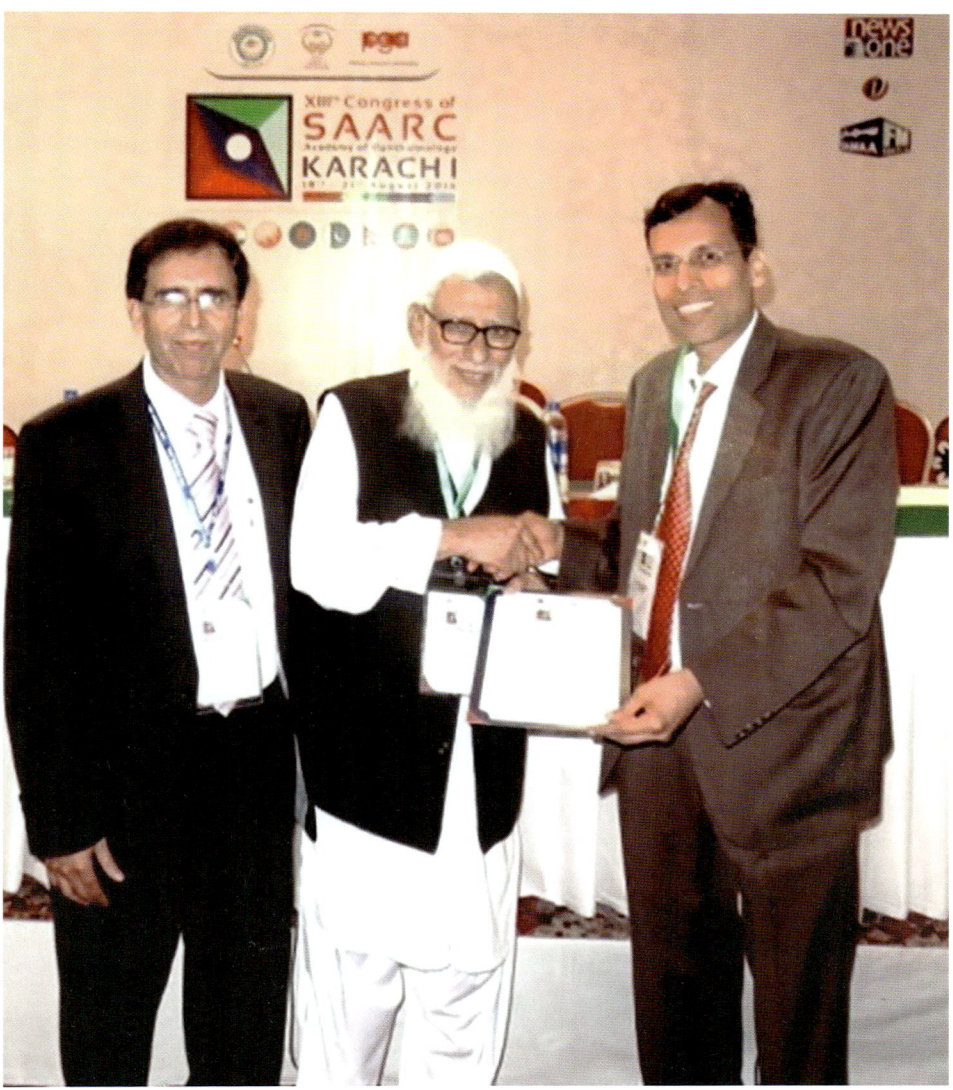

Figure 35. I received an award for best poster presentation during the South Asian Association for Regional Cooperation (SAARC) Conference held in Karachi, Pakistan, August 2016.

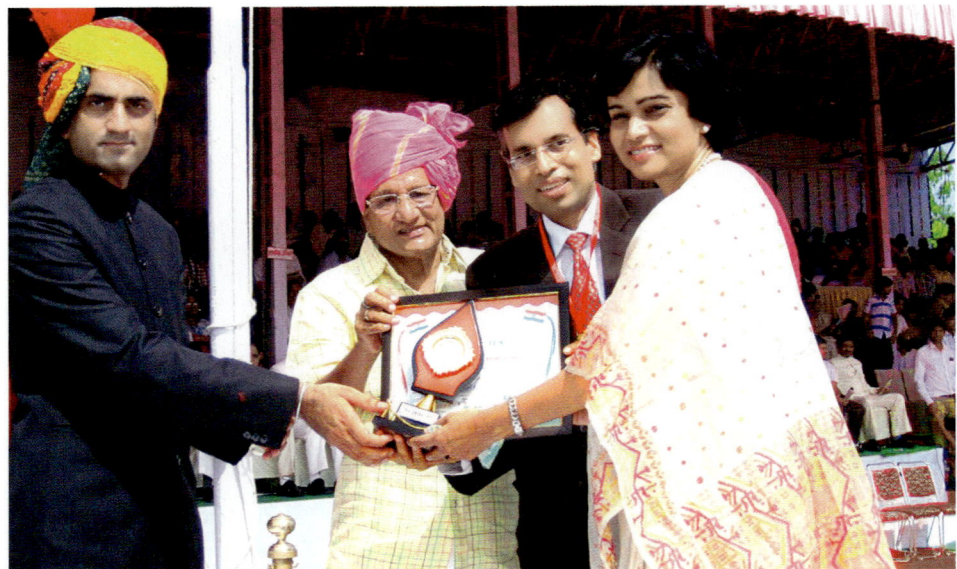

Figure 36. Dr Vidushi and I being honoured with an award in acknowledgment of our contribution to battling blindness by the Urban Development and Housing Minister of Rajasthan, Shri Shanti Kumar Dhariwal and District Collector, Kota, India, August 2013.

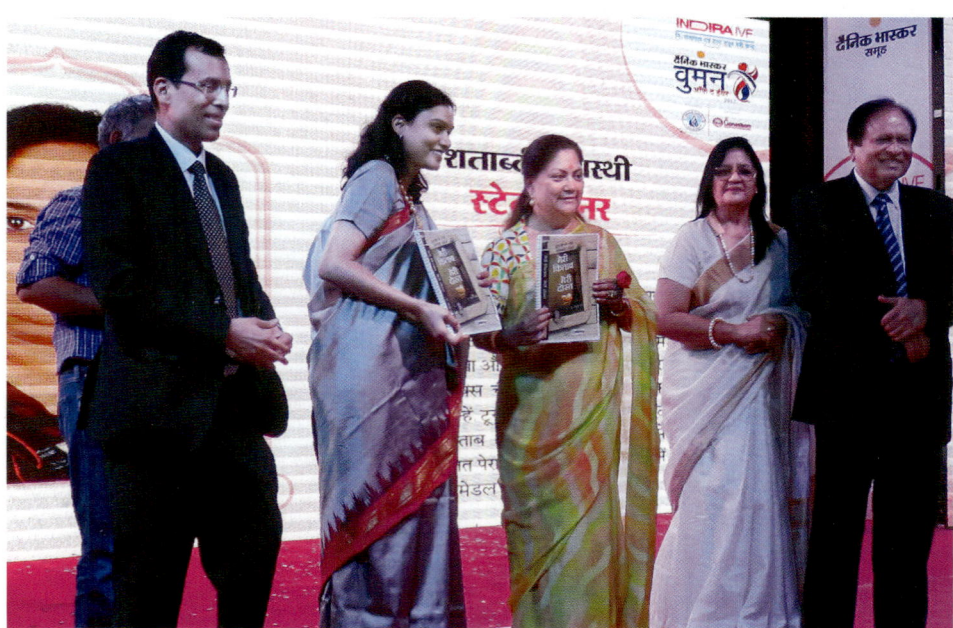

Figure 37. Chief Minister of Rajasthan Smt. Vasundhara Raje Scindhia unveiling Dr Vidushi's book *Meri Kitab Meri Dost* in Jaipur, June 2017.

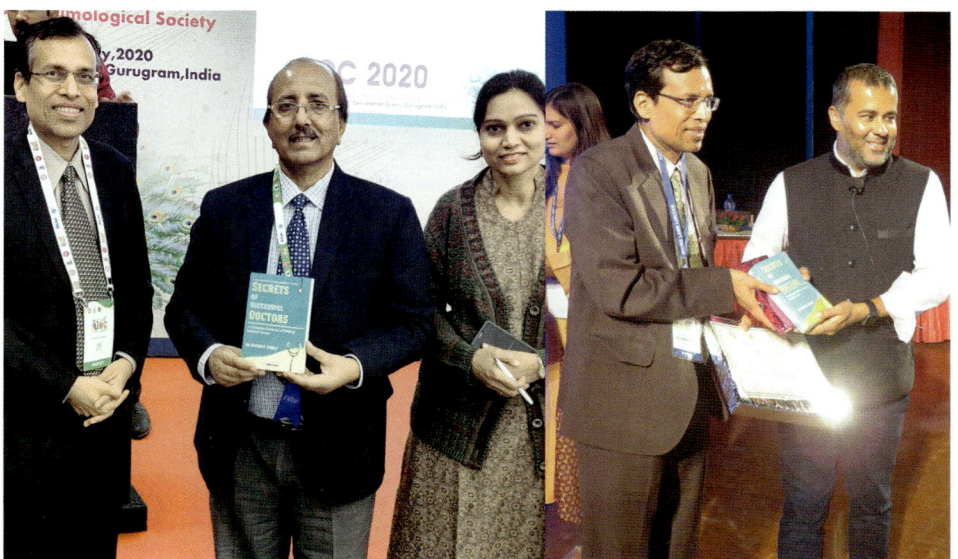

Figure 38. Left: I presented the book *Secrets of Successful Doctors* to my mentor, Padma Shri Prof. Jagat Ram (Director, PGIMER, Chandigarh), during the All India Ophthalmological Society (AIOS) conference in Gurgaon, February 2020. Right: I presented the book to famous author Shri Chetan Bhagat during the RAJMEDICON Conference, Jaipur, June 2019.

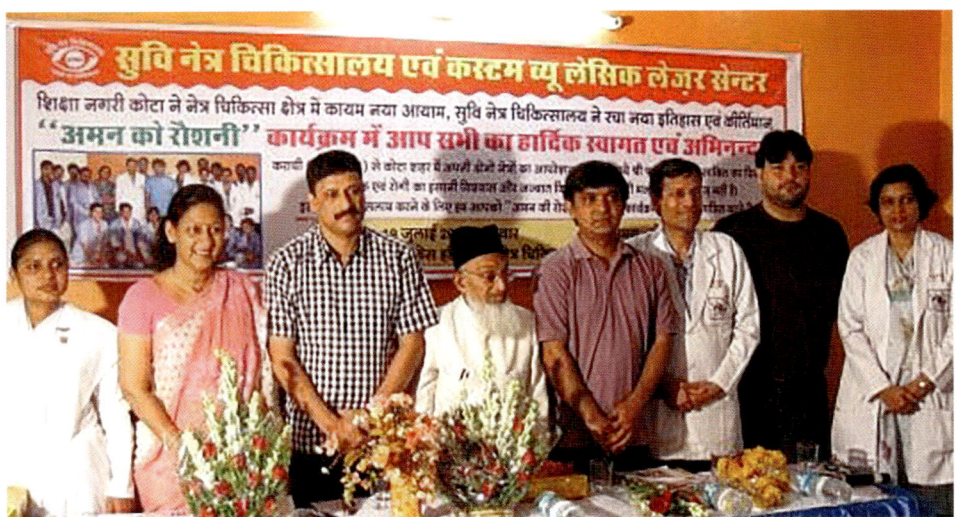

Figure 39. Mr Fahim Uddin together with his friend Mr Tokir Bukhari reached Kota from Karachi (Pakistan) for his eye surgery. Fahim Uddin underwent cataract surgery and implantation of Tecnis multifocal IOL at SuVi Eye Hospital. On 19 July 2012 a programme called 'Aman Ki Roshni' was organized at SuVi Eye Hospital Kota Conference Hall. Left to right: Brahmakumari Divisha, Mayor of Kota City Dr Ratna Jain, Inspector General of Police, Kota Shri Amrit Kalash, Shahar Qazi Shri Anwar Ahmed, Fahim Uddin, me, Tokir Bukhari and Dr Vidushi Sharma.

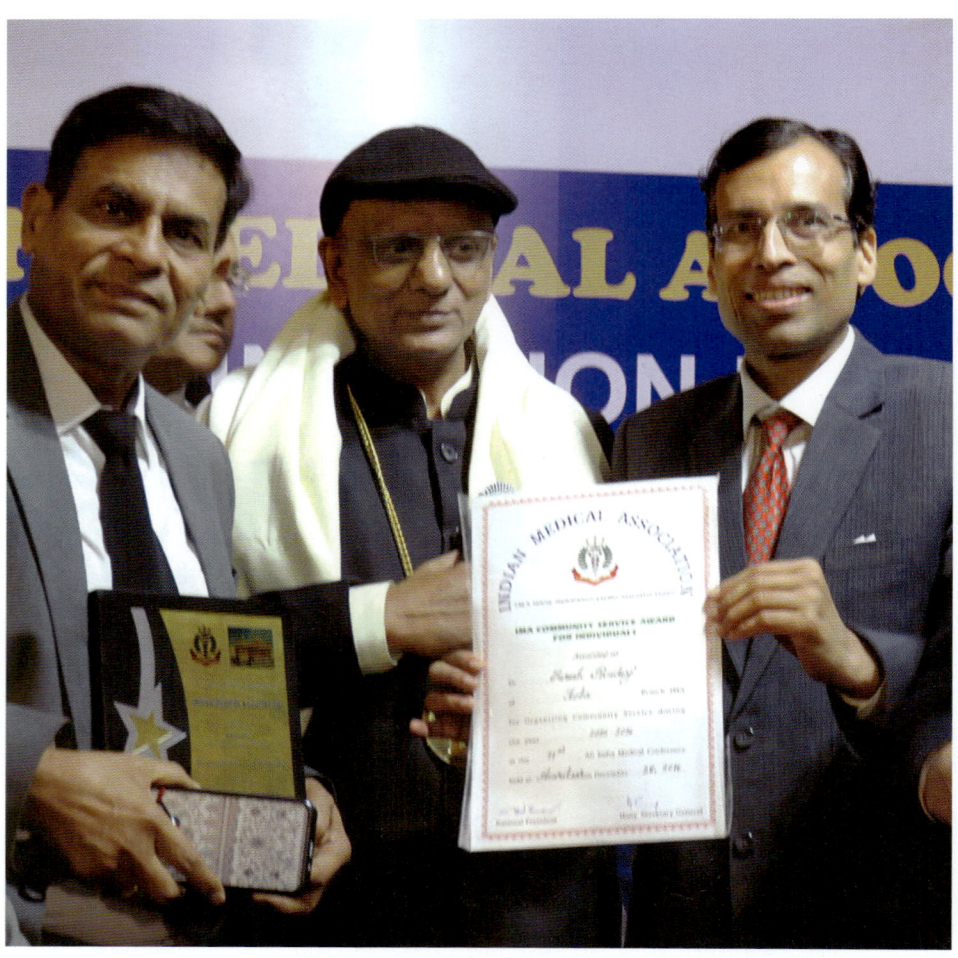

Figure 40. National President of the Indian Medical Association (IMA) Dr K.K. Agarwal honouring IMA Kota President Dr T.C. Acharya and me, the secretary, on the IMA Foundation Day at AIIMS, New Delhi, 7 January 2017.

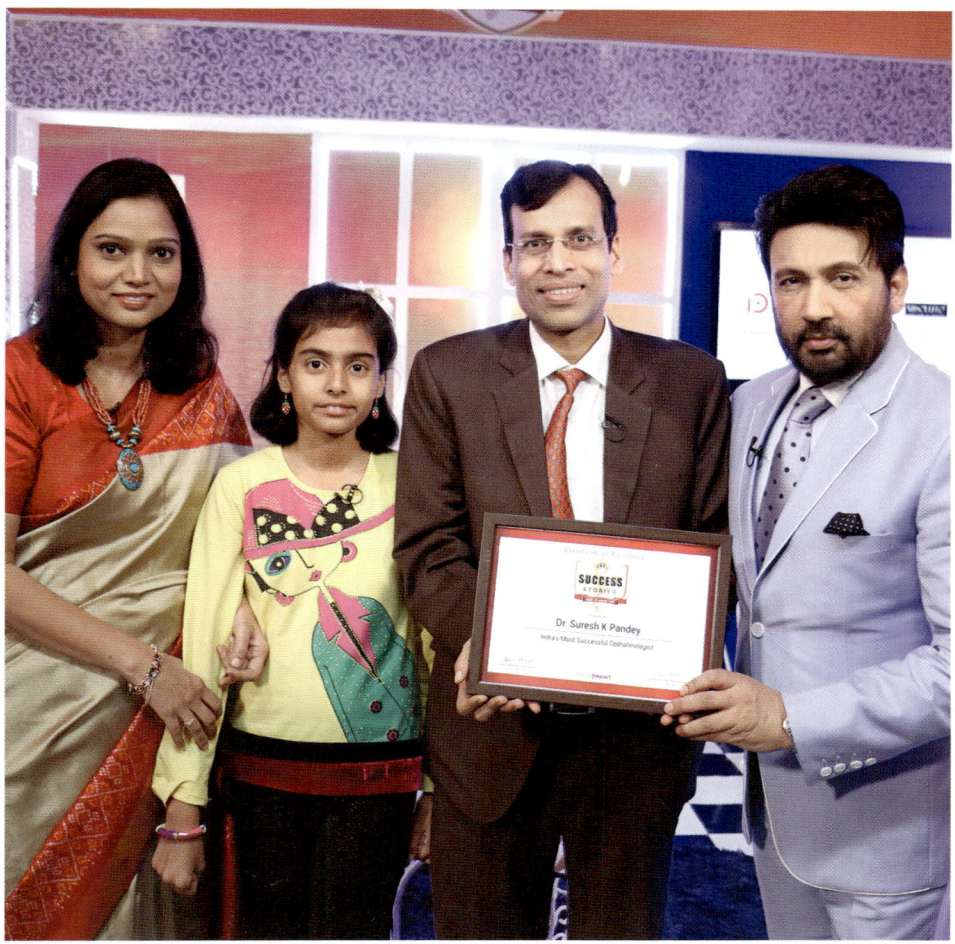

Figure 41. From left to right: Dr Vidushi, our daughter, Ishita Pandey, and I with film actor Shri Shekhar Suman in Mumbai during the *Zameen se Falak Tak* programme. This photo was taken during the shooting of the episode on the success story of SuVi Eye Hospital, Kota. It was broadcast on the national news channel Zee Business on 12 March 2017.

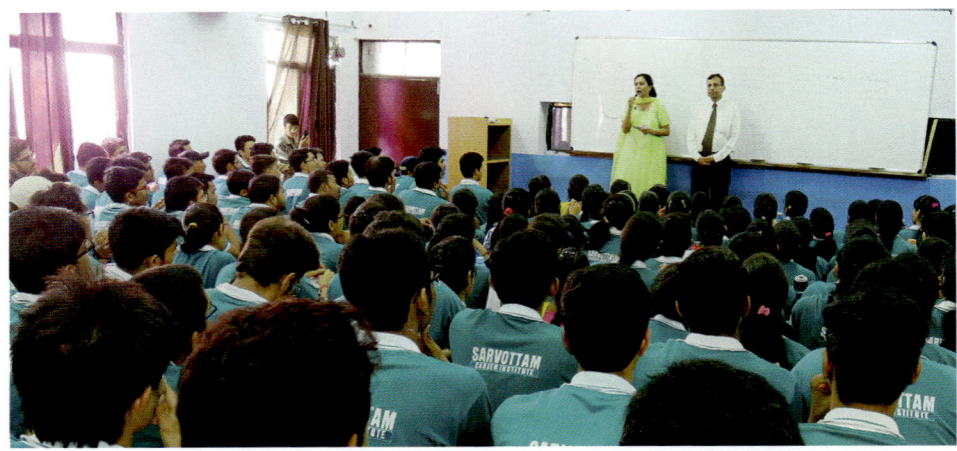

Figure 42. Dr Vidushi and I sharing our journey and the golden formula of our success with medical coaching students in Kota.

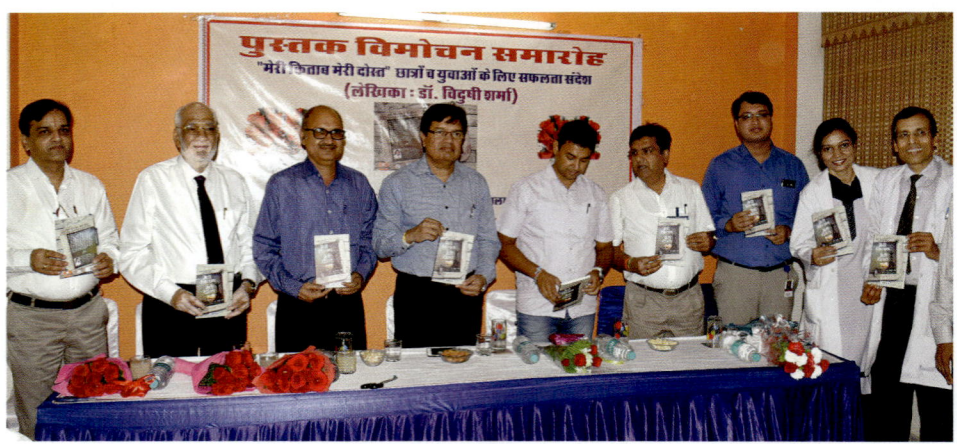

Figure 43. A motivational book for coaching students *Meri Kitab Meri Dost* was written by Dr Vidushi Sharma. The book was released on 12 August 2017, at the conference hall in SuVi Eye Hospital, Kota. (Left to right) Shri Govind Maheshwari (Director, Allen Career, Kota), Dr A.Q. Khan (Former Director, Rajasthan Health Services, Jaipur), Professor Pramod Tiwari (Former Superintendent, J.K. Lon Hospital, Kota), Professor Girish Verma (Former Principal, Medical College, Kota), Shri Rohit Gupta (District Collector, Kota), Shri Rajesh Maheshwari (Director, Allen Career, Kota), Shri Nitin Vijay (Director, Motion Career Institute), Dr Vidushi Sharma and myself.

to the hospital and discussed the problem with the gentleman. He asked me if I could see his wife at his home as she had diabetes, a slipped disc and rheumatoid arthritis. I agreed.

Meanwhile, I took a flashlight, proparacaine (an anaesthetic eye drop to relieve pain), antibiotics, lubricating eye drops, a bandage contact lens and fluorescein stain. After travelling about 10 kms, we reached their house and I could hear his wife crying out in pain. I asked her to open her eyes but she was unable to do so. I put one drop of proparacaine eye drops. After a few seconds, she felt instant relief and opened both eyes. I examined her eyes and found that she had a corneal epithelial defect with filaments in both of her eyes due to dry eye. I applied the bandage contact lens and her pain was relieved. I asked them to put lubricating, antibiotic eye drops and left. The gentleman visited me the next morning and thanked me profusely. I later found out that the gentleman was a senior reporter who spread the word about my services in his circle and the media.

This is how the first few weeks went: handling all emergency and routine cases that came our way. We never turned away anyone who visited our facility, even at odd hours. These cases were not attended to by any other eye surgeon due to odd timing and it was these patients who helped us gain popularity by word of mouth. We saw twenty-odd patients before deciding that perhaps our spontaneous plan would work out after all. But I was mistaken. Immediately after, we hit a roadblock.

One week later, the patients were merely trickling. We barely saw five patients a day and performed two surgeries a week, at best. The surgeries we did perform didn't pay well. For the cataract IOL surgery, the patient would pay us a partial amount. Sometimes, that was all a patient could afford; and sometimes, it was all the patient thought we should charge. 'If I wanted to pay ₹15,000 for a cataract IOL surgery, I would have gone to a surgeon with twenty years of experience.' Their words would sting but I learnt to not take offence. I accepted such patients as challenges and opportunities to create a bigger impact compared to other well-known eye surgeons in the city.

It was that horde of patients that was elusive. Some patients came in with grievances. Our hospital building was barely half a kilometre from the main road and several patients complained that it was difficult to locate the clinic. Patients were not coming to us, so we had to find a way to go to them. We decided to open an OPD clinic on the main road at Keshavpura. We rented this from another orthopaedic surgeon, Dr Nagesh Joshi. Dr Vidushi would be available for consultation at the Indra Vihar building and I would be available at the Keshavpura circle. All surgeries were conducted at Indra Vihar.

* * *

When I was in Australia, I thought that the hardest part of my job was performing surgery—which it sure is—but in Kota, I realized that running a hospital was no easy feat either. And to add to our stress, this job came with lots of free advice from our relatives. They shared their opinions with such conviction and confidence that it was hard for us not to listen. One advised us to join the famous charitable eye hospitals run by Lion's Club or Bharat Vikas Parishad. Another told us to offer a cut to anyone who brought us a cataract patient. There was no way we were getting entrapped in these unethical practices. We decided that we would continue to run our hospital at a slow pace. It was quite slow, because from the Keshavpura OPD, I would walk one kilometre to the Indra Vihar building repeatedly to perform the surgeries. It was significantly more time-consuming but we didn't have the money to buy a vehicle. But here, the same nagging relatives I was complaining about earlier, came to our aid. A distant relative left his scooter with us. The vehicle was ten years old; perhaps few would have been happy to acquire it, but to me, it felt like god's gift.

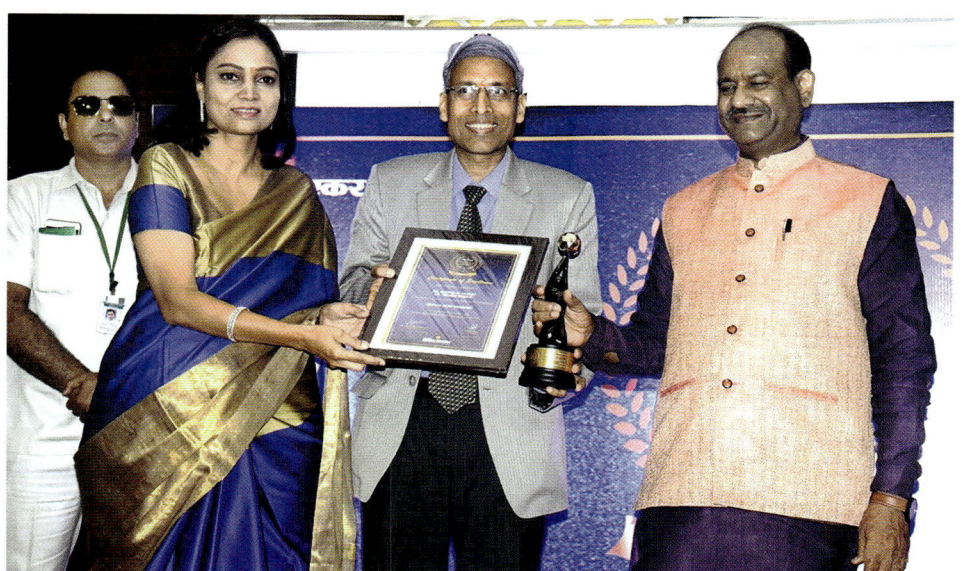

Figure 44. Current Lok Sabha Speaker Honourable Shri Om Birla presenting the *Dainik Bhaskar* Eminence Award to Dr Vidushi and me during an award ceremony, 11 September 2019. This award was in acknowledgment for our free eye surgery camps for needy children and increasing public awareness about ophthalmology and eye health.

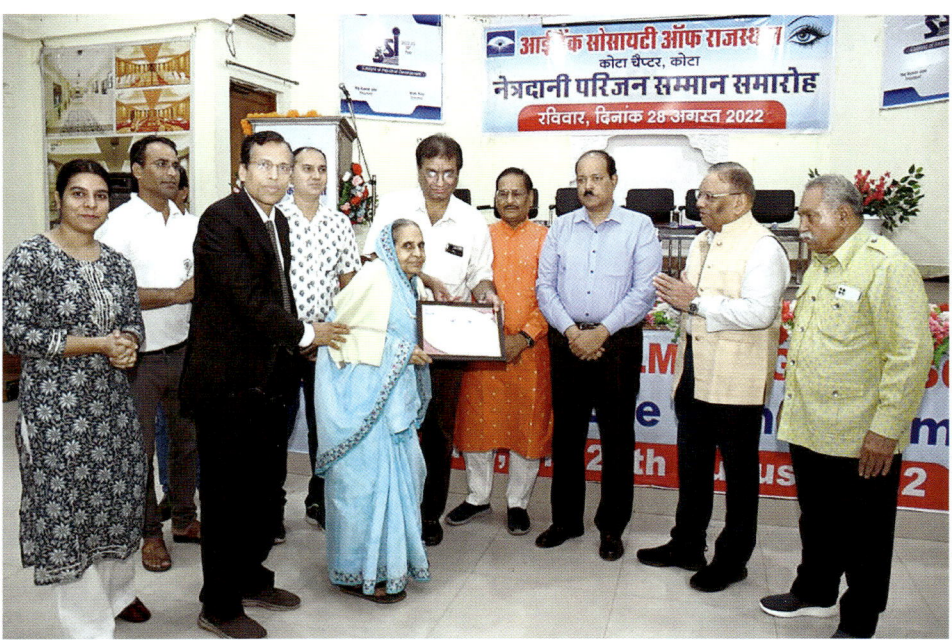

Figure 45. My father pledged for donating his eyes after his death and his wish was duly fulfilled. My mother Smt. Maya Devi Pandey was honoured during the Netradani Family Felicitation Ceremony, 28 August 2022. Left to right: Dr Shivangi Dwivedi, Govind Sharma, me, Smt. Maya Devi Pandey Dr Ashok Meena, Dr Vijay Sardana (Principal, Medical College, Kota), Shri Rajesh Birla, Shri Prasanna Kumar Khamesra (I.G. Police), Dr Krishna Kumar Kanjolia (President Eye Bank Society of Rajasthan, Kota Chapter).

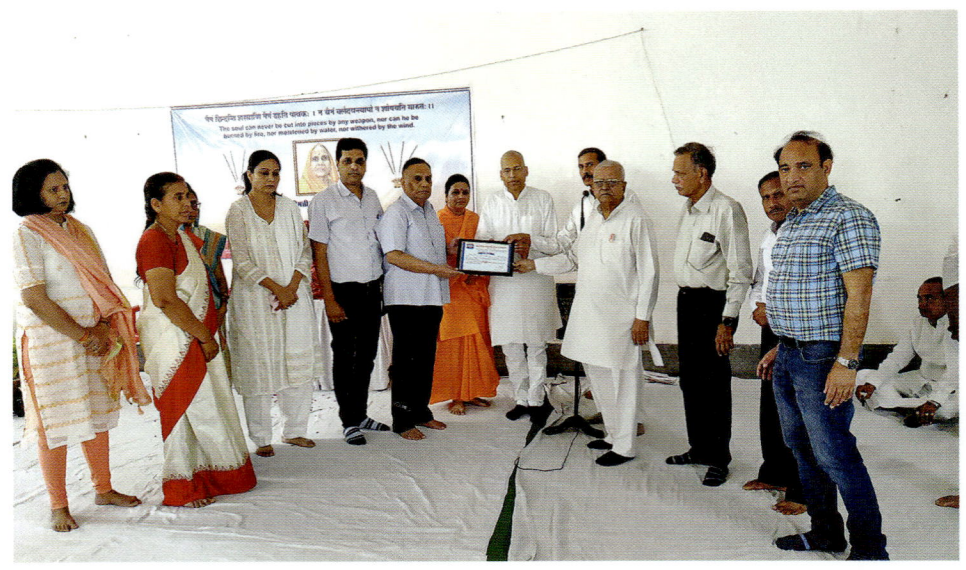

Figure 46. We fulfilled the pledge of donating my mother's corneas on 6 April 2023. During the tribute meeting on 8 April 2023, Eye Bank Society of Rajasthan, Kota Chapter honoured us with a certificate in appreciation of this eye donation. Pictured here (left to right) are Dr Anita Chauhan, Smt. Usha Pandey, Dr Vidushi Sharma, Dr Vishal Snehi, Dr K.K. Kanjolia, Sadhvi Hema Saraswati, me, Dr Rajesh K. Pandey, Shri G.D. Patel, Shri R.S. Paliwal, Shri Tarkeshwar Pandey and Shri Suresh Sedwal.

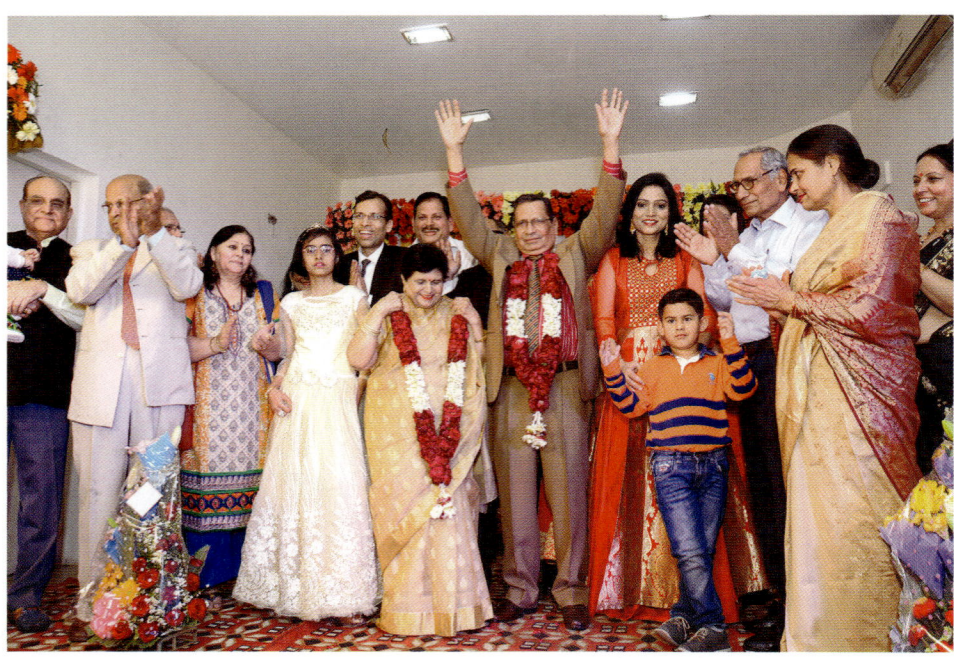

Figure 47. At the fiftieth marriage anniversary of my in-laws, Group Captain (Retd.) Shri K.M. Sharma and Smt. Sudha Sharma, 21 March 2017. Two months after this, my father-in-law left us for his eternal journey on 19 May 2017.

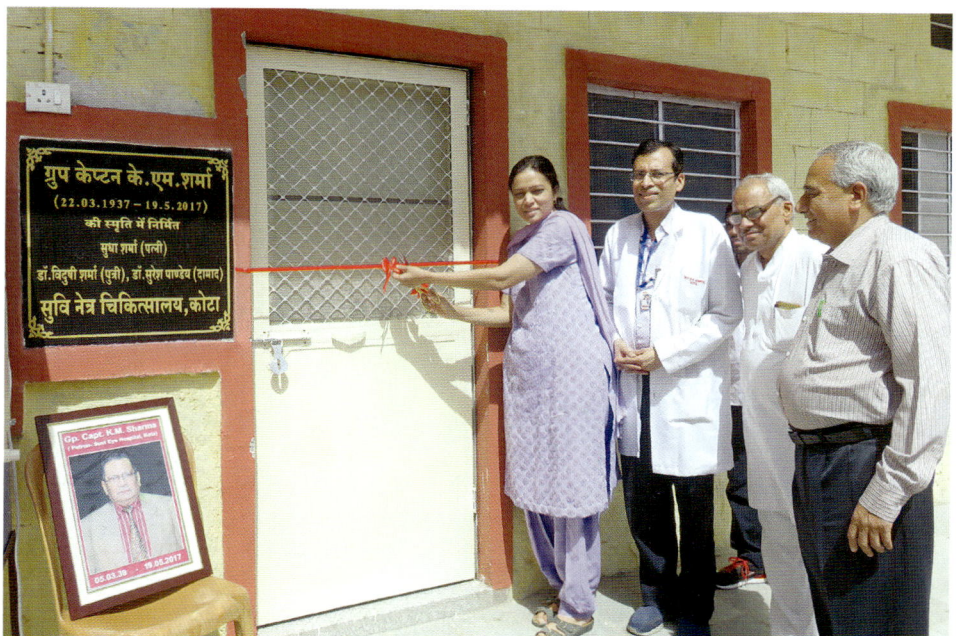

Figure 48. My mother-in-law donated ₹5 lakhs in sacred memory of my father-in-law to build a room in the Apna Ghar Ashram, Kota. Dr Vidushi and I inaugurated this room on 19 May 2019, on his second death anniversary.

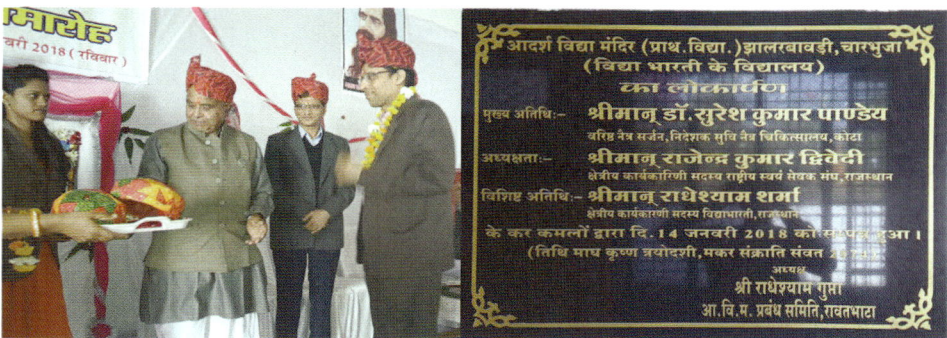

Figure 49. At the inauguration ceremony of Adarsh Vidya Mandir School, where I was invited to be the chief guest. Mr Rajendra Kumar Dwivedi, Mr Yogendra Gupta and Shri Radheshyam Gupta extend a warm welcome to me here.

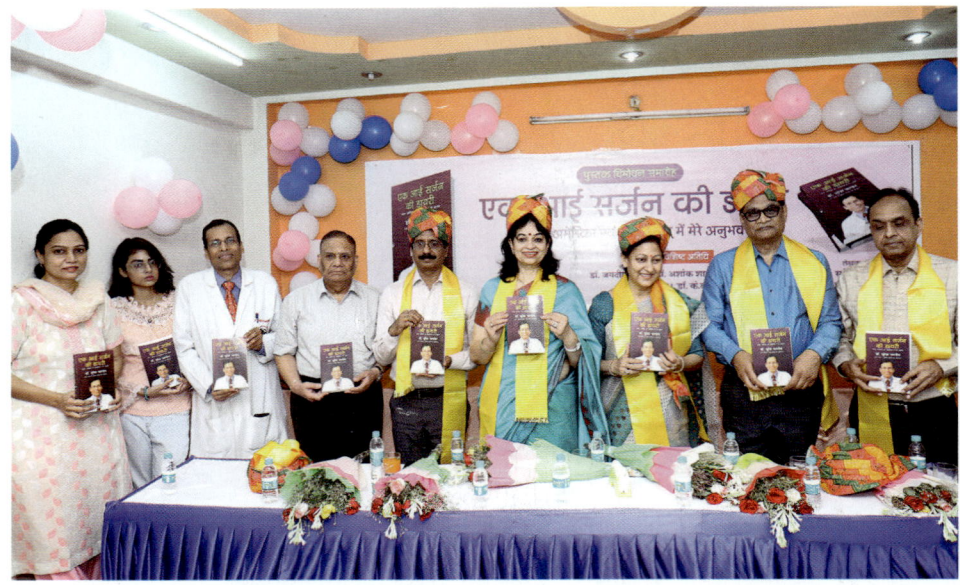

Figure 50. My memoir, *Diary of an Eye Surgeon: My experience in India, USA, and Australia* was released on 12 August 2023. Left to right in the photograph are: Dr Vidushi Sharma, Ishita Pandey, me, Dr K.K. Kanjolia (President, Eye Bank Society of Rajasthan, Kota Chapter), Dr Jagdish Soni (CMHO, Kota), Dr Sangeeta Saxena (Principal Medical College, Kota), Dr Ratna Jain (Ex-Mayor, Kota), Dr Ashok Sharda (Vice president, IMA) and Dr Girish Mathur (National President, API).

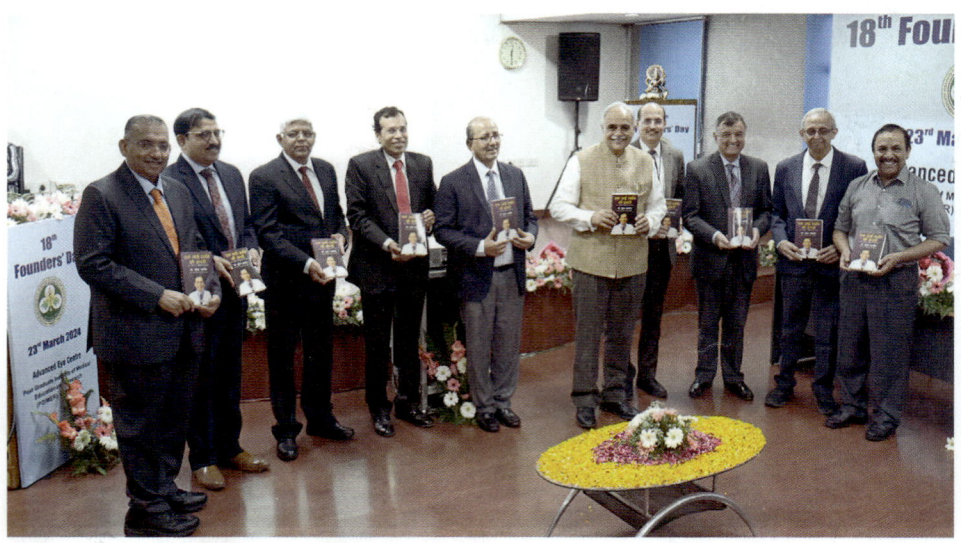

Figure 51. I delivered a talk on 'Save the Saviours' during the Founder's Day programme of the Advanced Eye Care Centre, PGIMER, Chandigarh on 23 March 2023. On this occasion, I also presented my book, *Diary of an Eye Surgeon: My Experiences in India, USA and Australia* to Dr Vivek Lal (Director, PGIMER, Chandigarh). Pictured here (Left to right): Dr Deepak Edward (Department of Ophthalmology, University of Illinois, Chicago, USA), Dr Parth Biswas (Vice President, All India Ophthalmological Society), Padma Shri Dr Amod Gupta, me, Padma Shri Dr Jagat Ram, Dr Vivek Lal (Director, PGIMER, Chandigarh), Dr S.S. Pandav (Chief, Advanced Eye Centre, PGIMER, Chandigarh), Dr M.R. Dogra, Dr Vinay Nangia and Dr G.R. Reddy.

## Bit by Bit

Despite our best efforts and now a scooter to run between our two centres, the flow of patients was scanty. The bills were piling on. In the first six months, we had earned ₹80,000 from surgeries and ₹20,000 from patient OPD fees. Our expenditure, counting rent, utilities, staff salary and other expenses like cleaning and maintenance, amounted to ₹1.25 lakhs. We had thought that if we cut down on our lifestyle, stopped going out for dinners or movies, we would be able to break even. However, we failed miserably. My father and father-in-law both offered financial help, but we asked them to wait. We had created this trouble for ourselves and we had to solve it.

Every evening, Dr Vidushi and I would sit with our account books and try to excavate new sources of funds. But no real solution would come to mind. Then one day, our account was credited with ₹2,00,000. It seemed miraculous but the miracle-maker was the government of Australia, who had sent us our tax refund. Whatever the source, we heaved a sigh of relief.

We were so pressed for cash that I didn't even think about travelling to participate in conferences. In Australia, every month, I would travel to participate in international conferences, but I couldn't do that anymore. And this worried me. Along with a successful career in the medical field, I had worked hard to stay active in academics and regularly participate in national and international medical conferences. I had presented research and clinical papers at several of these conferences. But now I realized that I had to prioritize and focus. The tax refund had allowed us to sail through for the time being and I wanted to ensure that we were never confronted with such a precarious financial situation again.

## Planning to Succeed

When I was in Australia, I read a famous book called *Put your Customers to Market your Business/Practice*. The book had a simple but profound message: ensure an outstanding experience for every customer so that they can become your brand ambassadors. I got this opportunity with Niharika Ghose, a student at Bansal Classes. She complained of experiencing intermittent headaches for a few months. I examined her and found that she had swelling in her optic nerves (known as disc edema). Optic nerves and retina are considered to be an extension of the brain; also why eyes are considered the window to the brain. While taking down her detailed history, she told us she had been taking Vitamin A supplements for the past nine months. I discussed her case with Dr Vidushi and we made a probable diagnosis of benign intracranial hypertension as a result of Vitamin A toxicity. An MRI scan of head confirmed our diagnosis and she was prescribed oral acetazolamide in consultation with a neurologist. In a few months, her swelling subsided and headache disappeared. Niharika was ecstatic—and she bore the good news far and wide across Kota. When I looked around, I saw many brilliant young students like Niharika, trying to build their careers. They all went to coaching classes near our hospital and would often drop by for an eye examination or with complaints of headaches. They studied for long hours and many had poor vision that needed correction.

It was Mother's Day on 14 May 2006. A sixteen-year-old student, Atul Sharma, was returning home from his coaching class. It was about 9 P.M. and as he was crossing a dark section in the street while talking to his family on the mobile phone, suddenly, someone threw chilli powder in his eye and tried to snatch his phone. Our neighbour, Rashmi Goyal, saw this as she was passing by in her car with her parents. She immediately stopped her car and challenged the robbers, who fled, and she conveyed Atul to our hospital. Dr Vidushi attended to him and started treatment immediately. After putting anaesthetic (proparacaine) eye drops, she thoroughly washed both his eyes and prescribed medicines, including lubricating eye drops. Atul recovered after two days. His mother came in after a week to thank Rashmi Goyal and Dr Vidushi for their help on the occasion of Mother's Day.

A lot of the coaching students had medical aspirations. They were deeply impressed with Dr Vidushi and my academic credentials. Most were surprised that we had decided to return to India, and that too to a small city like Kota. Dr Vidushi and I would often take time off to talk to them and motivate them. These students were very generous in spreading the word about us and our practice. Without our asking, they became our brand ambassadors. They liberally and enthusiastically talked about us and our hospital to whoever would listen, and slowly, at least within the student circle, we became a popular name.

If a patient came to us because of a reference, we ensured that they left after being given the best possible care. Around this time, we also hired more staff members who had to routinely call the patients whom we had treated and ensure that they were doing well. The patients and their families began to appreciate our caring and compassionate style of providing eye care. Our patients grew from five to ten per day. Soon, we celebrated one year of SuVi Eye Hospital. We had two reasons to celebrate: the first anniversary of our hospital and the fact that we had finally broken even.

## A Phone Call Away

I bought a cell phone in December 2005 and my mobile number was made public for any eye-related problem in Kota. It was something of an anomaly because most doctors would not share their personal number with the public. They wanted to avoid unnecessary calls—I circumvented the challenge by delegating my phone calls to my staff. And slowly, as the calls became incessant, I trained my staff members to receive and manage calls. On several occasions, I prescribed eye drops or tried to solve the problem of a patient who was sitting several miles away, over a phone call or text messages. Many patients sincerely appreciated our services, especially during the COVID-19 pandemic. Our trained team and I helped more than 10,000 eye patients over the phone (WhatsApp/video call) during the lockdown period. This became possible by effectively delegating work to our efficient team.

But this was not enough. I knew we had to do more to cement our place in Kota. Rumours were still rife. Many thought that we would wind up our business and leave in a month or two. Even Professor Billson had expressed his confidence in our academic capabilities, but not our business acumen. When we went to bid goodbye to him and his wife back in Sydney, he said, 'All the best, Vidushi and Suresh! I am giving you one year to try your new venture and if you are not successful in your mission, you are most welcome to come back to Australia and we will work together again.'

## The Power of Positive Perception

I remembered something else Professor Billson had told me—an advice I took to heart. He taught me the value of creating a 'positive perception'. I toyed with the idea for several days. How, I wondered, could we go beyond word of mouth and scale up? And, just then, as my eyes searched the room, I noticed the newspaper. Every morning, I read the *Dainik Bhaskar*, India's leading Hindi newspaper. *That's it!* I thought. *We need to get in the papers!*

Soon after, I got the opportunity. The media had covered our inauguration but we needed more. I started submitting articles to spread awareness, along with a few patient stories and how we had helped correct their eye issues. Over time, I built a rapport with journalists and editors and have now published over 200 articles with them.

What also made news were our efforts to help patients far and wide. We started a mobile eye care unit in March 2006 to offer affordable eye care to all nearby towns and villages. The unit bus was equipped with an auto refractometer, slit lamp and optical counter to prepare and dispense glasses. We supplemented this by organizing eye camps on days like World Health Day, World Sight Day, World Diabetes Day, World Glaucoma Week, among others. If a case turned out to be serious, we would ask the patient to visit our hospital for a complementary check-up. Slowly, our relentless efforts began to be highlighted in the media and played a vital role in creating awareness about our hospital and establishing our reputations as credible healthcare professionals in the region. But this didn't shield us from controversy that threatened to engulf everything we had made.

# 13

# A Tale of Caution

## Surviving Controversies

*'Often the difference between a successful man and a failure is not one's better ability or ideas, but the courage that one has to bet on his ideas, to take a calculated risk and to act.'*

—Maxwell Maltz

No one runs a successful enterprise without making mistakes. I was no different. Sometimes, I was shielded by luck but at other times, I wasn't. When I started performing cataract surgeries early in 2006, many patients would come to me with ultra-dense cataracts. No matter how much I wanted to avoid making large incisions for ripe cataract surgeries, I would eventually have to give in. These were not easy. Cataract surgeries in these cases came with an increased risk of corneal decompensation or a delicate membrane of the eye rupturing.

While my patients and I were lucky to never experience such complications, I did begin to notice moderate to severe corneal edema, leading to blurred vision for one week to ten days after surgery in some patients. I wanted to provide them with the best patient care I could and this wasn't it. I discussed this problem with senior eye surgeons and read extensively about possible solutions. I wanted to be proactive and regularly update my surgical methods. When I came across a solution, I immediately put it into practice. We started using newer phaco tips, sharper blades and dispersive viscoelastic solutions, and managed to resolve the problem before it reached gigantic proportions. But I wasn't always this lucky.

## The Eye Conference, a Controversy and Lessons Learnt

It was 2014. I was conferred with the prestigious IIRSI Gold Medal during the Indian Intraocular Implant and Refractive Surgery Society Conference held in Chennai. I received this award for outstanding work in the field of cataract surgery, teaching and international research. I used that opportunity to also launch my textbook and video atlas, *State of Art in Ophthalmic Surgery*. This textbook and video atlas were released by India's prominent ophthalmologists, Dr Keiki R. Mehta, Dr Amar Agarwal, Dr Lalit Verma, Dr Sudhank Bharti, Dr Kumar J. Doctor. After this conference, I returned home to Kota with a great sense of accomplishment. I felt validated and proud. But this happiness was short-lived. The next day at work, a patient brought me a vial of an eye drop (0.1 per cent nepafenac) that they had purchased from our pharmacy. This eye drop had been prescribed by one of our doctors to cataract surgery patients to minimize inflammation and pain. The gentleman told me to look closely at the packaging. 'Look at the manufacturing date,' he said, 'It says November 2014 whereas today is 8 July 2014.' I was shocked. I couldn't understand how this was possible.

I immediately called the vice president of the pharmaceutical company and brought this to his attention. I then submitted a complaint via email adding photos of the vial and our purchase bill from the company's authorized stockist in Kota. The vice president assured me that he would look into the matter and respond to me within twenty-four hours. Then a local delegation met with me and told me that it was a printing mistake. 'How could a printing mistake pass unnoticed through all your checking mechanisms?' I asked them. I could not believe it was a printing mistake as this was a very reputable pharma company. Why was this mistake not noticed and corrected? But the question was also applicable to us: why hadn't we checked? The truth is that pharmacists mostly pay attention to the expiry date. For the first time in my career, my attention was drawn to the manufacturing date. I asked them for a detailed explanation, but I wasn't given one.

Two days later, the news found its way into the local media under a controversial headline. Reading the news, drug inspectors arrived at our hospital for inspection. We showed them our bills and our complaints and thankfully, it convinced the drug authorities that we had no role to play in this fiasco. But they did suggest that we go to the police station and file an FIR against the supplier, the medical representative and the company. I was reluctant to file a police complaint but when they insisted, I complied.

The case was highlighted in the local media for three days with sensational headlines that called the eye drop counterfeit. It was an extremely stressful time. I thought this would affect our patient base and our reputation—it did cause worry among a few patients—but others came forward to report that the drops didn't lead to any adverse effects. But law had to take its course. A case was registered against the supplier, and medical representative and a trial was in progress. Our name was mentioned in the police inquiry. A few weeks later, a new case was filed against the supplier, company personnel and our pharmacist. We challenged this in the local court as an appeal. Our appeal was accepted and this case was dismissed.

Meanwhile, the pharma company was working on a thorough investigation and found that the chemical content of the eye drop was absolutely correct (0.1 per cent nepafenac). It really was just a printing mistake. Within a few months, the entire episode was dismissed. But all along, the fear of patients distrusting us or leaving our side was rife. I was deeply worried that this incident would tarnish our image. But thankfully, truth prevailed and our patients decided to retain their trust in us. It also taught us many lessons. First, we started getting most eye drops and medications directly from the company supply chain instead of local distributors. Second, we trained our pharmacist to inspect the box and accept only if the box is intact with the proper bill. We stopped accepting any supply that was not properly packed. We strictly followed the checklist and did a periodical evaluation to check and cross-check the protocol and checklist. All this was a very helpful exercise for us during the National Accreditation Board for Hospitals & Healthcare Providers (NABH) accreditation and also enabled us to confidently face our patients and tell them that we were careful and responsible healthcare practitioners.

There are hundreds of examples of hospitals going bust or doctors losing their reputations due to what is thought of as a singular unforeseen event. But what truly occurs is a slow breakdown of trust. This incident, in many ways, opened my eyes to the need to do better and do more. We were always careful about fostering and maintaining strong doctor–patient bonds but this particular incident encouraged us to rehaul our practices and ensure that we were doing everything possible to become the best healthcare facility. To do that, I had to lead by example.

One day, a fifty-year-old woman came to see us. She had lost her left eye to glaucoma—an eye disease involving high intraocular pressure. The other eye was controlled through three anti-glaucoma drops. But when the lady arrived, I could see that she often missed her doses. When I asked her, she complained that the drops caused redness in her eye and didn't improve her sight. I knew this was an excuse because these were trusted medicines that had treated many. It was important for her to understand that she couldn't skip her drops; it was also important for me that my staff understood that every patient was important and had to be given the best attention and care.

I asked the patient to close her eyes. When she resisted, I told her it was simply an activity we had planned for all patients. All they had to do was shut their eyes and do a few tasks. In a few minutes, the woman became extremely restless and gave up. 'I can't do it,' she said. And that's when I told her that she wouldn't have to stay in complete darkness if she continued to use her drops. The patient understood, as did my staff, that doctors don't just prescribe medicines, they must also talk to, explain and soothe the patient and offer holistic and complete healing.

## Valuing Feedback

As our practice grew, I kept the drug controversy and the scandalous news reports in mind. It motivated me to keep trying and revising practices and processes that ensured we always had our ear to the ground. This meant always paying attention to the patient's well-being but also their overall experience at the hospital.

As a young boy, I was always enthusiastic about writing appreciation notes as well as complaint letters. I thought why not introduce that system here? After all, one could uncover dormant or unmet needs by asking simple questions, or by taking feedback from patients on how to improve the services and gain competitive advantage through creative innovation. We started small with Hindi and English feedback forms which contained ten points, including availability of parking space outside the hospital, waiting time, experience at the reception during patient registration, experience of undergoing eye test (refraction), experience of being examined by the eye doctor, experience at the pharmacy, experience at the optical shop, and overall satisfaction. The form also included a blank space for people to write their suggestions. But unlike most feedback forms that never get analyzed, we made it a point to pay close attention to the feedback we were getting.

And that's how we caught one of our biggest problems. As our practice grew, we began to face the challenge of prolonged waiting time. This was a serious problem on Sundays or public holidays. On Sundays, our hospital was functional for half a day: from 9 A.M. to 2 P.M. But in these five hours, we sometimes saw fifty to sixty students as that is when many of them got the chance to see a doctor. Many other people would end up waiting for an hour. I was keen to resolve this problem but wasn't sure how, as no matter what, someone would have to wait. Then I came across feedback, which requested that students and the elderly be given priority on Sundays. I considered this and decided that it could be done. Based on this, the entire hospital staff was sensitized and trained to minimize waiting time for students and elderly patients on Sundays or public holidays. This move was appreciated by not only the student community, but also by the coaching centres of Kota. That day, I understood that running a successful practice needs equal parts caution and the humility to listen and act proactively. Additionally, it also needs empathy and a willingness to go beyond and bridge any gaps in the doctor–patient communication.

One day, a middle-aged zoology professor visited us for his cataracts. He underwent bilateral cataract-intraocular lens surgery at our centre with excellent postoperative results. A few years later, he visited us again, complaining of seeing floaters in front of his right eye. At that time, a visiting retina specialist, Dr Gunjan Prakash, used to come to our centre to examine patients with retinal problems. Dr Prakash examined him and informed him that he had a horseshoe tear (HST) in the retina of one eye, which needed urgent laser treatment to seal it and reduce the risk of developing retinal detachment.

A horseshoe tear is a special type of break in the retina, which can cause retinal detachment and loss of vision. Once a retinal detachment develops, the management is purely surgical and the results may not be very good. Both Dr Prakash and I explained to the patient his eye condition, the need for the retinal laser treatment and the risks involved. However, after asking numerous questions, he told us that he believed that visiting doctors were motivated by money and left saying he was unconvinced that he needed the treatment. This was quite an insult, especially because we take pride not only in our work and qualifications but also in the fact that we run a completely ethical practice and always advise to every patient only what is in their best interests.

But I also realize how frightening and disconcerting it can be for a patient to make a decision to undergo treatment. I smiled and recommended that the patient seek a second opinion. He visited us a few weeks later and told us that his vision was fine; he clearly didn't need treatment. A few months later, he visited again, suffering from a sudden drop in vision and we immediately knew that he had developed the retinal detachment. We resisted the 'we told you so' talk and told him that he needed immediate surgery. He successfully underwent the vitreo-retinal surgery and had a reasonable visual recovery. I often think about this incident—not because I want to prove myself right, but because I know that trust in medicine is still scarce. What is important is to not confront the patient or start an argument, but to be sure to document your diagnosis and your advice in detail. It's important to treat people with empathy and only because of our empathy did the patient feel comfortable enough to return. This is what builds patient trust, calms their anxiety and improves health outcomes—and no storming controversy can change that.

# 14

# Bringing Surgical Advancements to India

*'With confidence, you can reach truly amazing heights; without confidence, even the simplest accomplishments are beyond your grasp.'*

—Jim Loehr

In 1988, I went home for Diwali. I was looking forward to the few days of celebration—watching the illuminated night sky, walking around the colourful streets, and relishing the sumptuous food. It was a welcome break from my rigorous medical college study, lab work and assignments. After the Lakshmi puja, I accompanied my mother to meet a few relatives. It was going to be a quick visit but shortly after we reached one of their homes, I became a subject of ridicule. My aunt looked at my spectacles and said, 'Your eyes have grown weak at twenty? Look at me, I am fifty-eight and still have perfect vision.' My aunt knew that I was keen to study ophthalmology and she used that as an opportunity to berate me. 'If you cannot fix your own eyes, how will you treat others'?' What she said stunned me. I had never thought that my calibre would be doubted because of my personal eyesight.

I was immediately reminded of Dr José Ignacio Barraquer Moner. Practising in Spain, Dr Barraquer was always eager to improve classical procedures and experiment and use new surgical techniques. As early as the 1930s, he had pinpointed that the greatest challenge for him was to correct refractive errors by modifying the shape of the cornea. He was certain that the corneal curvature played a considerable part in determining the dioptric power of the eye. But his colleagues dismissed his thinking. They didn't think myopia or near-sightedness was something that needed to be corrected. Such eyes were considered healthy. All doctors had to do was prescribe spectacles and move on. There was one thing Dr Barraquer and my aunt had in common: they both didn't like spectacles.

Dr Barraquer argued that if any part of the body didn't function properly, it had to be corrected. It needed treatment. For him, spectacles were prosthetics, not a cure. So he set out to find a way to ensure a spectacle-free life to people. I deeply admired Dr Barraquer and his pioneering investigations. It was his work on surgically modifying the cornea that would eventually lead to LASIK treatments. But back then, there was no LASIK.

After the sting of my aunt's comment had passed, I channelled my inner Dr Barraquer. I promised myself that like him, I would work on the most innovative tools and technologies to help advance ophthalmic treatments. I preferred spectacles—they brought me a certain comfort and I didn't think I wanted to get rid of them. But I realized that many didn't understand the choice. It became clear to me that a lot of work had to be done to minimize the taboo associated with wearing glasses. But, this doesn't mean that those keen to get rid of glasses don't have access to the latest technologies. I decided that a balance was overdue. When I became a doctor, I stopped bothering about these negative comments but I would be frequently asked why I, an eye doctor, wore spectacles. I wore them so that people understood that there was nothing wrong with wearing glasses. It was my choice. But I was also prepared to offer them the best care if they decided to get rid of their spectacles.

One day, a middle-aged couple came rushing to see me. It was after 8 P.M. and I didn't have any new appointments scheduled. But as they were already at the hospital, I decided to see them anyway. The man said that his daughter was going to get married the day after tomorrow but there was one major problem. I was confused. 'But she can't wear her spectacles and get married,' the woman said. Despite the seriousness of the situation, I laughed. At the most unusual hour of my workday, in the unlikeliest fashion, I was faced with the most common problem. Patients often came to us to buy contact lenses or correct their eyesight not because they wanted to but because society expected them to. Umpteen young women had come to me to get their eyesight corrected because they feared rejection from potential suitors and in-laws.

I sat the parents down and told them to stop worrying, to stop looking at spectacles as a taboo. When the bride-to-be arrived, I told her to not worry about the society's approval. 'Society is all of us,' I told her. 'Together, we can change the mindset of our people.' But they had made up their minds. Nothing I said could alter that. 'All right,' I finally said. I asked the young woman if she would like to wear contact lenses to her wedding. She nodded. I ordered a pair of lenses and asked my staff member to train her on how to use them. The staff also explained the need for carefully removing contact lenses before sleeping. Crisis averted, the family left happily.

A few weeks later, the young woman returned. She was suffering from contact lens-induced keratitis. She had worn her contact lenses to the wedding but shortly after, her right lens had fallen out and got lost. The woman was terrified of losing her left lens so she had kept it on day in and out. The result was a corneal infection in the centre and a corneal vascularization in the periphery. Her eye had developed ulcers. Four weeks of intense treatment followed and only after that, could we save her eye. We had seen another case where an eye was lost due to a severe infection and I didn't want the situation to repeat itself at any cost.

Over the years, I had seen a few such cases that reiterated the importance of awareness and patient counselling. But sometimes, despite our best efforts, we are unable to make a difference. There's an overwhelming demand for LASIK laser refractive surgery. And sometimes, it's for the right reasons, such as people whose professions depend on perfect eyesight. And that's what motivated me to try LASIK after spending years wearing spectacles. I decided that perhaps it was time to try it out for myself. I imagined a spectacle-free life and its obvious advantages while performing surgery.

Most of the time, our own thinking makes us weak or strong. '*Ladki paraya dhan hai, paraye ghar jawegi*' (The girl child is never one's own, she'll be married off into a different household). This is an oft-repeated line by parents and grandparents. We often see that females often themselves pose the biggest challenges to the progress of their gender. When a boy and his family go to a girl's home seeking a matrimonial alliance, senior female members of the boy's family sometimes inspect the prospective bride very carefully and pass comments like 'she wears spectacles', 'she's too thin', 'she has dark circles under her eyes', etc. People label bespectacled women and mock them. Like the case mentioned above, I have seen several cases where girls leave their contact lenses in and do not remove them, leading to corneal ulcer.

Uncorrected refractive error is the second common cause of preventable blindness or visual impairment. According to the studies, 30 to 50 per cent of such victims are female. Even today, we encounter such cases. In February 2019, the SuVi Eye Hospital team was invited to set up an eye check-up and spectacle distribution camp at Government Girls' School, Talwandi, Kota. When I was distributing the spectacles, I came across two cases. The mother of one girl came up to me, touched my feet and requested me to prescribe some medicine for her daughter since she could not be allowed to wear spectacles.

Another girl was myopic with minus 10 dioptres power in her eyes. She sat in the front row and struggled to finish her work after a lot of scolding, just because she could not see clearly. She asked her parents many times about the need for glasses but they told her to eat a healthy diet and gave her eye drops that they hoped would correct her vision. Her mother told me that spectacles were a taboo in their family, especially for girls.

According to the published studies, barriers to spectacle compliance include scarring on the nose, poor appearance, fear of injury, lack of parental investment in correcting the medical issue, negative attitude of society toward those wearing spectacles, etc. The face is part of the identity of people, and women and girls in particular are made to feel much more conscious of it. A girl wearing spectacles is not given fair consideration in matrimonial alliances. Spectacles are seen as a marker of weak overall health. There is no single reason for it—the entire mindset of the society, the impact of the family perception, and the self-image of women and girls, all have a role to play. Women empowerment, thus, is key to tackling preventable blindness of this nature. According to author Steve Maraboli, 'The empowered woman is powerful beyond measure and beautiful beyond description.'

* * *

In May 2000, I was invited to Belo Horizonte in Brazil to speak at an ophthalmology conference. During one of the sessions, I met a heavyweight LASIK surgeon, Dr Fernando Cançado Trindade. He invited me to visit his eye institute (Instituto de Oftalmologia Cançado Trindade), containing all the latest equipment. While showing me the LASIK operation theatre, he asked me about the power of my spectacles. I told him that my spectacle power was minus 3.5 dioptre and he assured me that he had helped several doctors to get rid of their glasses and he could correct my refractive error through LASIK. But when my eyes were investigated, we found that my corneal thickness was 580 microns and my intraocular pressure was 22 mm of Hg. With the borderline intraocular pressure (IOP), it was first necessary to evaluate the cause for it and so the decision to perform LASIK laser refractive surgery was postponed.

My cornea was on the thicker side. However, I have also seen hundreds of patients with high refractive error (minus 8 diopters or more) with a thin cornea (thickness less than 500 microns), in whom it is not possible to perform LASIK laser refractive surgery. Many such patients were very uncomfortable with high-powered glasses and wanted to get rid of them either due to reasons like marriage or job or other personal issues. I realized that here was an opportunity—there must be millions who can't correct their eyesight because of thin corneas or very high refractive error. I decided to pay close attention to inventions that could help them. It would take almost a decade for me to realize this dream. In 2011, we introduced LASIK laser refractive surgery in Kota by installing the NASA-approved VISX CustomVue LASIK Laser machine, micro-keratome unit and a VISX WaveScan wavefront aberrometer. It was a hefty investment that cost us about ₹3.5 crore, but it was the need of the hour. Using this machine, not only could we perform LASIK surgeries easily, and the perfect outcome also motivated to popularize some other techniques that were less known in our city and this part of India during 2010–2017. These included phakic lens implantation, premium intraocular lenses (toric, trifocal, expanded depth of focus, trifocal/multifocal toric implants) and piggyback lens implantation, zepto nano pulse technology, etc. to manage difficult adult and paediatric cataract cases.

The Invention of the phakic lens was especially close to my heart because it could correct high refractive errors in patients with a thin cornea. I had seen the journey of LASIK and now with the invention of the phakic lens, I wanted to introduce the same joy to the patients like myself. I got my first opportunity with twenty-two-year-old Harsha Banthiya. Harsha was a B. Tech final year student who had myopia since early childhood. Her spectacle power was minus 7.5 dioptre together with minus 2.5 dioptre cylinder. She was a basketball player competing at the state level. She was now training to play at the national level and had always found it difficult to wear glasses while playing, so she was seeking a solution. She had consulted several ophthalmologists in Kota, Jaipur and Indore, but had been unable to rid herself of spectacles. LASIK Laser Refractive surgery was not an option because she had a thin cornea. When she came to me, I examined her eyes closely and suggested the most recently available option: Toric Implantable Phakic Contact Lens (Toric IPCL).

Until then, the phakic lens (known as Implantable Collamer Lens, manufactured by STAAR® Surgical's) was the only expensive option that at the time, cost around INR 92,000 for both eyes. The ICL would take a few weeks to arrive and it was available till minus 20 diopters refractive error. It was not possible to pass the benefits onto patients of high myopia with a high cylindrical power of more than 20 diopters. But I knew we could bring this cost down by increasing awareness and making an alternative phakic lens to help thousands of such patients of high myopia. I discussed this with Care Group, an IOL manufacturer in Vadodara, to come up with a less expensive phakic lens. They managed to bring down the cost to roughly around INR 62,000 at the time for both eyes. Harsha's operation was a very big deal. Not only was she going to be India's first patient to receive such an implant, she would also be the first to use an Indian-manufactured toric IPCL.

When she came in for the surgery, I helped her relax and assured her that the operation would be successful. I then used an anaesthetic eye drops to numb her eyes. I made a side port incision and injected a viscoelastic (viscous) solution in the anterior chamber of the eye. After this, it was time for the main incision. The phakic lens was loaded in the cartridge and then implanted in the ciliary sulcus of the eye. It was directed on the iris plate without touching the cornea or the crystalline lens. The entire surgery took ten minutes. Shortly after the surgery was complete, Harsha regained vision of 6/5 (and N5 for near) unaided from both eyes.

## Making Eye Care Affable, Available and Affordable

A twenty-eight-year-old software engineer, Sridhar Gopal, had consulted several prestigious eye institutes in South India but had not been able to fulfil his dream of being free of his glasses. After watching several of our videos on YouTube, he planned a visit to Kota. His power was minus 21 dioptre spherical and minus 3 dioptre cylindrical (180) in the right eye and minus 23 dioptre spherical and minus 2.25 dioptre cylindrical (180) in the left eye. The STAAR ICL (Implantable Collamer lens) was not available in such a high power to correct his myopia. After a detailed check-up, we planned for the toric implantable contact lens to correct his myopia. He underwent the procedure first in the left eye and then the right, after which he completely recovered his vision.

## For the First Time Ever: Zepto-rhexis in a Five-Month-Old

Another time we brought the best of world ophthalmology to India was when five-month-old Yanhavi Shukla was suffering from congenital cataract in both eyes, was brought to us. Her father was an engineer at the Bhabha Atomic Research Centre, Mumbai, and her mother was a homeopathic doctor. The couple consulted a few eye doctors in Mumbai, who told them that lens implantation could be done when she turned ten. Her father, Vikram Shukla, had undergone cataract surgery and Toric lens implantation at our hospital. Vikram called me in May 2017 and asked me if he could bring his daughter to Kota for cataract surgery and lens implantation. After getting a positive response from us, the couple came to Kota. I examined the child thoroughly and we decided to perform cataract surgery with IOL implantation in both eyes. Performing the capsulorhexis in infants (children less than one year) remains challenging due to the very elastic anterior lens capsule and low scleral rigidity. I used 'Zepto nano pulse technology' or 'Zepto-rhexis' (a device manufactured by Centricity Vision, USA that was introduced to our practice recently, for the first time in Rajasthan) to perform the capsulorhexis. The surgery was performed in both eyes and the child regained her vision immediately after. She became more active and responsive and her parents' joy knew no bounds. Paediatric cataract was my thesis topic and I was glad I could help. I published several papers on this topic and also wrote a book on Paediatric Cataract Surgery, as mentioned before.

## India's First Tecnis Toric IOL Implantation

A fifty-eight-year-old railway engineer from Mumbai, Praveen Bhatnagar, was suffering from poor vision in the left eye for the past five years. He had age-related lenticular changes as well as corneal astigmatism (1.68 dioptre) and was very keen to regain vision without having to wear spectacles. After a comprehensive examination, I suggested the implantation of AMO Tecnis Multifocal Toric intraocular lens. This was the first time that such a lens was implanted in India—and at 75 per cent of the cost that a procedure like this would have cost in a metro city. Praveen regained near-perfect vision and would only require spectacles to read very fine fonts.

Over the years, we have successfully managed to treat about 1.5 million patients and performed more than 100,000 complex and routine eye surgeries, which include oculoplastic, eye trauma, vitreo-retina, cornea transplantation as well as LASIK and cataract surgery with premium intraocular lens implantation. Every day at the hospital, we reinforce our motto of 'Competent Care with Compassion'. But the credit for this success only partly goes to me; the real heroes, mavericks and doers are my entire team, without whom even a single feat is unimaginable.

# 15

# It Takes a Team

## Growing Together

*'There is no such thing as a self-made man. You will reach your goals only with the help of others.'*

—George Shinn

## When Our Staff Become Santa Claus

It was Christmas 2006. One of my staff members, Anirudha Sharma, read the news about a nearly blind child, Anil, in a tenement area of Kota. His father was an alcoholic and his mother worked as a daily wage labourer. She had to leave her son at home, so she would lock him in the room or tie him with iron chains. One day, the neighbours learnt about this and informed the media. The news was published with a sensational headline but what Anirudha gleaned from it was that the child had very poor vision in both eyes. As a result of this, possibly, he had delayed progress and cerebral palsy-like symptoms. He asked me if we could help and I immediately agreed.

Anirudha left and brought the child and his mother to the hospital. I examined his eyes and found that he had total cataracts in both of his eyes. We advised a paediatric check-up and treatment so his systemic condition would also improve. After a few days, we performed cataract surgery and artificial lens implantation in both eyes. The child's life was transformed. The family received some help from a local NGO and he was admitted into a school. I was thankful to Anirudha for his idea. That Christmas, he was Santa Claus.

Soon, SuVi Eye Hospital and Lasik Laser Centre was two years old. We had expanded our practice from seeing ten patients a day to 250. But in 2006, Dr Vidushi and I were not just entrepreneurs, we were also parents to our daughter, Ishita. Ishita filled our lives with love and laughter but she also made me acutely conscious of my role and responsibilities as a father and doctor. For the first time in my life, I was in a position to mentor and give back, and I was keen on making the most of the opportunity.

As the workload increased, we kept updating our medical equipment to ensure that patients received nothing but the best treatment. Our hospital made sure that there was no compromise when it came to patients' services and care. But as people sought us out, I realized it was time to recruit qualified staff members to help us manage them more effectively. I had learnt about successful teamwork from observing symphony orchestras and sports teams. If you go to a symphony performance, you will notice how excellent individual musicians and a talented conductor work together with precision. It's primarily because they are driven by the same vision. The conductor produces no music himself, but achieves that vision by directing others.

I realized that running a hospital was not much different. Managing doctors can only realize their vision through the motivation and coordination of everyone else involved in the practice. The result can be harmonious or discordant, pleasing or stressful, depending upon the skill of the conductor. While hiring the best doctors and staff is an important step, I learnt that it's not just about hiring the best players, but also those who can work together with others and spur them on to achieve their optimum. There may be opportunities for solo performances, but the focus must be on what can be achieved as a team. The perfect example of team work was shown during the Live Surgery event of the 44th Rajasthan Ophthalmological Society Conference (ROSCON) hosted by the SuVi Eye Hospital & Lasik Laser Centre, Kota.

## Hosting Live Surgery – 44th ROSCON 2022 Conference

In August 2022, we took up the responsibility of hosting the Live Surgery event of 44th annual conference of the Rajasthan Ophthalmological Society (ROSCON 22) at the SuVi Eye Hospital & Lasik Laser Centre. It was a herculean task, which could only be managed by a very efficient team. I held a meeting with my team members and asked for their suggestions. Everyone was ready to work hard to make this event successful and memorable. Our team worked day and night to paint and renovate the entire hospital premises and operation theatre. The event was held on 14 October 2022. Several renowned eye surgeons performed live surgery at the operation theatre of SuVi Eye Institute & Lasik Laser Center, Kota, which was telecast at Hotel Menaal Residency, Kota. The surgeons who performed live surgery included Dr Mukesh Sharma (Entropion surgery), Dr Ajay Aurora (Anti VEGF injection), Dr Amulya Sahu (sub-2 mm SICS surgery), Dr Sheetal Mahuvakar (Pterygium with autograft with fibrin glue), Dr Partha Biswas (Phaco with Johnson & Johnson Eyhance IOL), Dr Arun Kshetrapal (Phaco with Hoya Nanex IOL), Dr Virendra Agarwal (Phaco with Johnson & Johnson Synergy Toric IOL), Dr Suresh K. Pandey (Phaco with Zydus Sifi mini well IOL), Dr Sonu Goel (Phaco with Hoya Vivinex Toric IOL), Dr Mayank Agarwal (Toric IPCL Phakic Lens), Dr Saurabh Luthra (Phaco with Alcon PanOptix IOL), Dr Prateek Gupta (Phaco with Adtec Comfort IOL) and Dr Pankaj Sharma (Phaco with Johnson & Johnson Synergy Toric IOL). Our staff team members were praised by Dr Partha Biswas (Chairman, Scientific Committee, All India Ophthalmological Society), Dr Amulya Sahu and other doctors during the inauguration ceremony, for their teamwork. Dr Vidushi and I thanked and celebrated all the team members and their families for the excellent job they did.

## The SuVi Eye Family

We feel proud to say that most of our staff members have been working with us since they started their careers. We are blessed to have excellent team of doctors: Dr Satyendra Kumar Gupta, Dr Deepesh Chhablani, Dr Nipun Bagrecha, Dr Vidushi Sharma and myself. Our excellent team members (also known as the SuVi Eye family) include Arun Gautam, Vishnu Rathore, Govind Sharma, Sandeep Sharma, Bajrang Meghwal, Devraj Suman, Bhupendra Soni, Gauri Revani, Roshni Singh, Aishvarya Sharma, Satya Prakash Sharma, Kuldeep Gurjar, Rajesh Gupta, Bhupendra Gautam, Shrikant Sharma, Sandhya Suman, Vinod Verma, Vishnu Sharma, Ramesh Potter, Ranjana Rathore, Narendra Meghwal, Bharti Verma, Kapil Chopdar, Monu Bairwa, Yashwant Bairwa, Kanika Sharma, Praveen Malav, Ramavtar Sharma, Pallavi Agarwal, Muskan Tahilyani, Harishankar Prajapati, Himani Shrivastava, Jagdish Paswan, Ramdev Yogi, Omesh Rathore, etc. Each of our team members worked hard on the personal front to groom their personalities as well as on the professional front to improve their working capabilities. Regular classes were conducted and motivational books were given to SuVi Eye family members for personality development. Below are two interesting stories.

## Using His Own Eye Treatment as Motivation to Help Others

There was a school near our hospital's Indra Vihar centre. One day, I saw that a staff member, Bajrang Meghwal, was rubbing his eyes vigorously. When he stopped and opened his eyes, I saw that they were bloodshot. I immediately asked him to come to the hospital but he refused. He told me that he had seen several doctors but had not got permanent relief. I assured him that we would try our best to get him lasting relief and convinced him to see us.

In the evening, he arrived with his mother, who told us that his job was in danger. He had been working as housekeeping staff in a school but due to the persistent redness of his eyes and his deteriorating vision, he was unable to see clearly and do his job properly. No doctor had been able to help him effectively. He and his family members were very worried.

Dr Vidushi examined his eyes carefully. After averting the eyelids, she noticed he had giant papillae, known as cobblestone papillae, that were causing the redness. He also had a central posterior sub capsular cataract in both eyes. Dr Vidushi first tried to regress the cobblestone by administering a supratarsal injection in both eyelids. She also told him to use ice-cold compresses four times a day and stay away from dust, sunlight and other pollutants that could aggravate the eye allergy. Within forty-eight hours, there was remarkable improvement in the itchiness and redness of his eyes. Half the battle was won.

We now had to treat his cataract. We evaluated his eyes thoroughly, conducted a few tests, and suggested that a multifocal lens would be most suitable for him. His younger brother was working at Allen Career Institute at the time, whose medical officer, Dr Sanjay Soni, approached us and said that he would arrange for the rigid poly-methyl methacrylate (PMMA) intraocular lenses, free of cost for him.

Bajrang was only twenty-one. Implanting a rigid PMMA IOL would need us to enlarge the corneal incision from 2.8 mm to 6.5 mm and he would become dependent on spectacles for near and far distances. We wanted to avoid that, so we declined Dr Soni's help. Instead, in order to finance the operation, we allowed them to pay for one-third of the operation costs in a manner that suited them. Appasamy Associates, too, helped us by offering us a free lens. His surgery was successful and Bajrang regained perfect vision. The experience left an indelible mark on him. He told us that he would really like to work with us at the hospital. We accepted.

In June 2006, he joined our team as one of the first OPD assistants. He was a keen learner, attuned to the details. Slowly, he learnt how to record vision, how to use an auto-refractometer, how to note the pressure using the non-contact tonometer (NCT) machine, how to dilate the eyes for retinal examination, and how to explain medications and other precautions to postoperative cases. Bajrang showed great drive and tenacity. In his free time, he would watch educational ophthalmology videos on YouTube. Now he is also planning to complete a certification to become an ophthalmic technician. Bajrang has been on this journey for the past seventeen years. Today, he is our star multitasker—adept at IOL power calculation, optical coherence tomography, oculus pentacam, specular endothelial cell count, fundus photography, Humphrey visual field examination, patient counselling, and many other tasks. He also edits our social media photographs and videos. When Mahesh Gupta, his former boss at Shiv Jyoti senior secondary school, sees him now, he is thrilled at Bajrang's incredible journey from a janitor to a key member of SuVi Eye Hospital.

It is people like Bajrang who make the hospital what it is. It's easy to hire people with great qualifications, but it's better to hire someone who is passionate, hungry to learn and keen to lead a purposeful life. When people know their purpose, they can turn their life around. As Viktor E. Frankl writes in his book *Man's Search for Meaning*, 'A man's deepest desire is to search for meaning and purpose'. That's the kind of culture we've built at the hospital—where the team members are supportive of each other, well-trained, understand the expectations and respect the fact that we're all working towards a common purpose.

## Master Troubleshooter

Like Bajrang, we also have Vishnu Rathore. Previously a newspaper delivery person, Vishnu is now the right-hand man of Dr Vidushi. At the age of twenty, he joined SuVi Eye Hospital and learnt how to assist Dr Vidushi in the OPD and in the operation theatre, as she did oculoplastic surgery and LASIK laser refractive surgery. She taught him about managing the entire team, as well as maintaining the entire building. Vishnu worked day and night to supervise the herculean task of renovating the operation theatre and some parts of the building a few weeks before the Live Surgery event during the 44th Rajasthan Ophthalmological Society Conference that was relayed and telecast from the operation theatre of our hospital.

As our team was growing, we ensured that key team members had the authority to make important decisions on their own within the framework of the overall plan. This helped develop a sense of trust among our staff. It has helped them function efficiently as well as bring creativity and initiative to their work. A lot of times, employers want a lot from their staff but offer little in return. We tried to be mindful of our staff's expectations by ensuring they are rewarded and that they are provided with a flexible and adaptable work environment. Perhaps that's why when we were dealt a challenging card, our team was ready to help us face it with a stoic, unwavering mind.

After three years of running the hospital, we were assured of our practice and were confident that we could build a long-lasting institution in Kota. Dr Vidushi and I decided that it was time to move into our own building. After one failed attempt, we were back to our search for a plot. Most properties were over our budget. Finally, we found a plot in the Talwandi area. It was merely half a kilometre away from our Indra Vihar location. The plot had a small house on it, but both the house and plot had now been put on sale. Still, there was a problem. The house was situated at T-junction and was numbered the unlucky number 13. Many buyers had considered this property but after finding out about the T-junction and number 13, which they considered its 'Vastu Doshas' (inauspicious according to Vastu Shastra), did not move ahead with the purchase.

We did not believe in these superstitions. When we contacted the owner, he was happy to sell his plot to young doctors. It turned out to be a smooth deal. This time, our balance sheet and income tax return files were in order, and the bank agreed to give us a loan to cover 75 per cent of the cost. We purchased the land with the house in May 2009. Six months later, the construction began. It was scheduled to finish in one year or by December 2010 but eighteen months in, the project was nowhere near completion. Every day, I would chase the contractor to finish the work. One day, he abandoned the project and ran away.

We were shocked. We had spent a crore rupees on it already and by now, getting another loan from a bank seemed impossible. We tried our best but failed to find another contractor to complete the pending work. We had no idea what to do. What was worse, the contractor decided to assert legal force against us. We consulted our lawyers and did our due diligence—we now needed to show that we were staying in the building to avoid its seizure. So in April 2011, I shifted into the half-finished building. There was electricity and water, but no fans or working toilets.

Dr Vidushi and I had to come up with a plan. We identified our two staff members, Vishnu Rathore, Mukesh Mohit and put them in charge of the construction. We gave them the responsibility of finding reliable construction workers and getting the work done. Dr Vidushi planned the next steps and supervised their work. She made a list of everything that had to be done: laying floor tiles, false ceiling, water connections, painting, among others. I was fully focused on operating on the patients and ensuring their satisfaction. Both Vishnu and Mukesh assisted Dr Vidushi and devoted themselves to getting the work done. They would reach the construction site at 8

A.M. every day and stay till 8 P.M. After three gruelling months, the building was ready.

We inaugurated the new hospital in July 2011 and were inundated with patients. Viral conjunctivitis had spread across Rajasthan. One of our old patients also came in for a consultation. He was among the people who had warned us about the effect of 'T' and Vastu Dosha. 'Wow,' he now said, looking around, 'it looks like this is the reverse T effect.' The building was not yet complete but the reception was fully packed with patients. Vishnu thus proved himself the backbone of our hospital. He told us, 'Don't worry, I will fix all the pending work'. Dr Vidushi was the proudest mentor, admiring his incredible career arc from being a newspaper delivery person to OPD/OT assistant to building manager.

When I look back, I realize that the success of the hospital is owed to our hardworking and passionate team members. We certainly set up the processes—from early adoption of technology to offering the best surgical procedures—but without the commitment of team members and leaders, we wouldn't have managed to come this far. The success of the hospital today rests on their shoulders.

# 16

# Breaking the Glass Ceiling

## The Journey of Dr Vidushi Sharma

*'The true republic: men, their rights, and nothing more. Women, their right, and nothing less.'*

—Susan Anthony

It was 10 April 2003 and I flew from Sydney to San Francisco to participate in the ASCRS Conference. Flying over the Pacific Ocean, I wondered about the life of the surgeon who was going to be honoured at the conference. I was going to witness a historical event: the introduction of Dr Daniéle Aron-Rosa to the Hall of Fame at the ASCRS. The brilliant contributions of Dr Aron-Rosa have made cataract surgeries easier for ophthalmologists around the world.

Born in France in 1934, Dr Aron-Rosa studied physics before turning to medicine. She received her medical degree in 1962 at the University of Paris, completed her residency at the Hopitaux de Paris Assistée Publique, and a fellowship at the AP HP University of Paris. Her interest in physics sparked her interest in ophthalmology which she then chose as her specialization. It was then that she saw how early ruby lasers had very slow pulses. Immediately, Dr Aron-

Rosa saw that she could use her physics background to create a faster laser pulse, specifically for retinal and cataract surgery.

But, as with many women doctors, scientists and inventors, her work was shrouded in conflict. It was assumed that Dr Aron-Rosa's first pulsed YAG Laser was a direct descendant of the Krasnov Pulsed Ruby Laser, when it wasn't. She had to invent new technology to deliver a non-invasive laser incision. She won many awards for the invention of the YAG laser after she achieved this and became the only woman to be included in both the ASCRS Ophthalmology Hall of Fame and also received the Charles Kelman Innovators Award in Ophthalmology. But more importantly, she inspired young women around the world to pursue the untrodden path of ophthalmology. And one person taking direct notes from her life, was my wife, Dr Vidushi Sharma.

Dr Vidushi completed her MBBS as well as Ophthalmology residency from the country's premier medical institute, All India Institute of Medical Sciences (AIIMS), New Delhi. When I asked her why she chose ophthalmology, she said because it offered her the adrenaline rush associated with performing delicate sight-restoring surgeries and the flexibility to not have to deal with stressful life-and-death situations. But none of this has been easy for her. When Dr Vidushi joined as a senior resident at AIIMS, New Delhi, the unit handled oculoplastic surgeries. Every week, patients who suffered from droopy eyelids, acid or chemical burns around the eye, or eye or eyelid cancer would arrive from across North India.

She did not, however, get the opportunity to perfect her sight-restoring surgical skills there as she'd usually end up handling only oculoplastic cases. Years later, when Dr Vidushi and I started our own hospital, she finally got the opportunity to hone her skills.

Fourteen-year-old Ashok Suman had noticed pain and redness in his eyes. This would lead to recurrent headaches and blurring of vision in his left eye. Then he lost vision in his left eye completely. When he visited a doctor, they told him he had inflammation (uveitis) in both eyes, as well as glaucoma in the left eye. There was nothing they could do. Young Ashok, they said, would have to live his entire life with vision only in one eye. But at least the right eye could be saved. The doctor performed glaucoma filtering surgery, called trabeculectomy, in his right eye to control the high intraocular pressure. Despite the surgery, the vision in the right eye kept deteriorating. Ashok was depressed and suicidal. The fear of blindness is extremely common and Ashok was feeling the full weight of it. It was then that Ashok came to SuVi Eye Hospital. Dr Vidushi examined his eyes and saw that he had a complicated cataract with 360-degree irido-lenticular adhesion. This had reduced the size of his pupil and led to glaucoma.

Dr Vidushi examined his case and planned for cataract surgery and IOL implantation in the right eye. There was an additional complication of very high intraocular pressure in the right eye, which could lead to permanent loss of vision. The surgery was planned after a lot of discussion and deliberation. Dr Vidushi planned to use the Ahmed glaucoma valve, a special device used for treating complicated glaucoma cases, to control the intraocular pressure. She started the surgery by injecting a peribulbar block in the right eye to anesthetize it. Then she made a side port incision in the cornea and injected a dispersive jelly-like substance inside the space between the cornea and iris to cover the delicate corneal endothelium. A blunt spatula was used to separate and gently break the tiny adhesion between the iris and lens. These adhesions had developed due to repeated inflammation and had prevented the pupil from dilating even after putting strong dilating eye drops. Since it was almost impossible to remove the cataract through a small (4 mm) pupil, Dr Vidushi used special nylon hooks to dilate the pupil to 8 mm.

After achieving satisfactory pupillary dilatation, she stained the anterior lens capsule with trypan blue dye and made a circular 5 mm opening in the anterior capsule. Finally, she used the phacoemulsification machine and performed phaco aspiration to suck the soft cataractous lens using vacuum. After this, she removed the cortical fibres from the capsular bag of the eye. Close to completion, Dr Vidushi noticed a thick plaque on the posterior capsule. She decided to remove the plaque to help maintain a clear visual axis. This was followed by the loading and implantation of a hydrophobic acrylic foldable intraocular lens. The surgery took ninety minutes in all and Dr Vidushi thanked God as the cataract IOL surgery was completed uneventfully.

But all was not yet done. She still had to perform another surgery to implant the Ahmed glaucoma valve to control the high intraocular pressure in the right eye. This was our hospital's and Rajasthan's first implantation of this valve. Dr Vidushi made a blunt conjunctival dissection at the supero-temporal quadrant of the eye. She gently inserted the valve under the scleral flap and put the silicone tube of the valve in the anterior chamber. One and a half hours later, when the surgery was finished, the right eye was patched. As the patch was removed the next day, Ashok screamed with joy. He had regained his vision and in only seeing the eye, it had improved from hand movement to 6/12 after surgery. His wide grin was infectious and the entire hospital celebrated with him.

I congratulated Dr Vidushi on the fantastic surgery and was appalled at how gender discrimination threatened to suppress someone as brilliant as her. Her excellence, I could tell, was a result of her own entrepreneurial initiative and in spite of no support and encouragement from her male peers. It reminded me of the quote by Gloria Steinem, 'A woman without a man is like a fish without a bicycle'.

'If one considers published reports, over half of female trainees report experiencing discrimination within the operating theatre and when in theatre, felt they received less autonomy than male colleagues,' Dr Vidushi once told me. To add to this, she is vocal about how there's an 'old boys' club' mentality, which discourages female trainees from participating more actively. Research shows that almost 40 per cent of women physicians work part-time or leave medicine altogether within six years of completing their residencies. What can change this? Dr Vidushi believes that women need to come forward to reverse this trend.

Social media can be employed as an effective tool to try to increase the visibility of women in surgery. It already has. In 2015, #ILookLikeASurgeon Twitter campaign encouraged female surgeons to post pictures of themselves to challenge some of the persisting gender stereotypes within medicine. In 2017, ASGBI's women in surgery group launched #HowIBecameAWomanInSurgery, designed for women surgeons to share their experiences during surgical training. The WinS forum has its own Facebook page and Twitter feed. In April 2019, the #ChangeTheNorm campaign encouraged participants to discuss and debate issues in surgery and challenge stereotypes of a 'typical surgeon', to welcome greater diversity. Encouraging women surgeons to consider leadership opportunities is another way to support their career development and improve the visibility of senior role models.

My conversations with Dr Vidushi are always centered around hope and improvement in the industry. She often says that after every storm, the sun comes out, sooner or later; that the reign of female inequality in medicine is slowly, but surely, reaching its end. As newer generations of women continue to populate our medical school classrooms, hopefully she will get to see a time when the expectation is that when someone comes in to see a physician, they find a woman, not a man in the doctor's chair. However, the reality is that many patients have certain reservations about women doctors. While they may trust women more and think they have greater empathy, some patients also feel that female doctors are not as competent. But Dr Vidushi has always faced difficult situations head-on, strengthened by her training at AIIMS as well as the University of Sydney. This ensured that she could do a variety of ophthalmic surgeries—not just cataract-lens implant surgeries, but also LASIK laser refractive surgery, oculoplastic surgery, glaucoma surgery, squint surgery, routine and complex ocular trauma and so on, which cannot be performed by most ophthalmologists.

There are many initiatives to ensure that women healthcare professionals form their own groups in order to ensure good mentoring and career progression. Dr Vidushi has been at the frontlines of this effort. She has delivered several lectures at the Indian Medical Association (IMA), contributed articles and worked to strengthen the women's wings of the IMA. Sub-specialties are also forming women's societies, like the Women in Ophthalmology Society, which has affiliated chapters in other parts of India, like the Women Ophthalmologists' Society (WOS). What women doctors need are tools and opportunities to advance their professional growth. And that's what Dr Vidushi tries to give them through greater interaction with women colleagues. At SuVi Eye Hospital & Lasik Laser Centre in Kota, she conducts regular sessions for young ophthalmologists, including women, about the career options and unique challenges of women ophthalmologists.

Dr Vidushi has excellent speaking and oratory skills. She provides the voiceover of most of our YouTube videos. I encouraged her to deliver talks during ophthalmic conferences and IMA meetings. Her speeches have been appreciated by medical professionals and have attracted several doctors to visit Kota for learning and fine-tuning their skills.

She has also been at the forefront of providing quality care to all patients, irrespective of their capacity to pay. Always willing to go the extra mile, she has examined over 50,000 patients in the eye awareness camps and performed several free surgeries. I have watched her speak at various public forums with pride and receive several awards like the 'Women of the Year Zonal Award' from the former Chief Minister of Rajasthan, Vasundhara Raje. But I know that the day when she will be the Doctor or the Person of the Year is not far.

## Dr Vidushi's Advice to Young Doctors

- Focus on getting the best possible training at the earliest opportunity. This is even more important for women, as it becomes very difficult to devote time to full-time rigorous medical training programs at a later stage in life, particularly after marriage and kids.

- At an early age, it is possible to travel far and wide for the best training opportunities, especially in surgical disciplines. Medical practice is not easy because of heightened patient expectations and a fast-spreading aggressive consumer culture. In such a scenario, it is absolutely essential to get the best possible clinical training, so that your competence is your biggest strength when starting a clinical practice.

- Choose your work based on your own personality and preferences. Some people are very good at communication and interpersonal relations and therefore do well in private practice. Some other people are interested in teaching and do well in an academic setting. Some realize that they would do well in non-clinical branches and some others decide they want to change their field altogether.

- Assess your priorities and desires and make an informed decision, as you can't keep changing your mind. The most important thing is to define success for your own self and then stick to it, to be truly happy.

# 17

# One Lakh Surgeries and Counting

## The Journey of a Left-Handed Eye Surgeon

*'Nothing splendid has ever been achieved except by those who dared believe that something inside them was superior to circumstance.'*

—Bruce Barton

Lata Agarwal, fifty-eight, a native of Nagda, MP, had severe difficulty in lying supine on her bed due to morbid obesity, cardio-pulmonary issues and Meniere's disease (a disorder of the inner ear that can lead to dizzy spells or vertigo, and hearing loss). In 2009, she started noticing extreme deterioration in vision and consulted several eye doctors, but none were able to help her. Lata found it impossible to lie flat on the operation table. Almost five years passed, her cataracts matured and she lost vision in both her eyes completely. She consulted more than a dozen ophthalmologists in various cities, from Indore to Chennai to Ahmedabad, but doctors would clearly refuse to perform the surgery because of her inability to lie on the operation table.

One day, Lata heard about me and visited SuVi Eye Institute & Lasik Laser Centre. I examined her eyes and took stock of the challenge in front of me. And then I decided I could handle it. I took her to the operation theatre and made her sit on a plastic chair. Another plastic chair was used to support her legs. I performed the phacoemulsification surgery of the left eye while Lata sat. It was an extremely challenging surgery because of the unusual position but I was determined to do it. I extracted the cataract and implanted foldable Multifocal Tecnis IOL (22 D) in her eye—the surgery was complete in ten minutes. This was perhaps the world's first case of topical phacoemulsification and Multifocal IOL implantation performed on a seated patient. The patient regained complete distance and near vision (6/6 and N6) without any glasses. And it was done by a surgeon who was told he didn't have a surgical hand and binocular three-dimensional (3D) vision.

## Struggling to Learn Eye Micro-surgery

There was nothing more challenging for me than learning micro-surgical skills. It requires several important functions, the ability to move your instrument within a small space of 3.5 mm, surgical dexterity to use both hands and both feet, and great hand–eye coordination to achieve perfect precision. As one can imagine, the eye is a small organ (2.5 cm) and any slight mistake or movement can lead to permanent damage, which may cause visual impairment or even blindness. During phacoemulsification, a surgeon needs to use their dominant hand to hold the phaco handpiece and non-dominant hand to hold the second instrument (chopper). They need to use one foot to focus the operating microscope and the other to press down the footswitch of the phaco machine. It is like driving the world's most precarious car. If it's challenging for right-handed doctors, it was nearly impossible for me as a left-handed one. Most of my seniors were right-handed, so if I had to learn, I had to copy the surgical steps of a right-handed person with my left, which was catastrophic. Some instruments of eye microsurgery were also designed with right-handed surgeons in mind. It was like getting stuck in a world where no one spoke your language.

When I joined PGIMER, Chandigarh, in January 1995, I was called to cover an emergency corneal transplantation. It was a winter night and the winds were howling outside. Professor Jagjit Singh Saini was performing the transplant. The opaque (diseased) cornea was removed and replaced with the donor (transparent) cornea. In order to fixate the donor cornea, fine 10-0 nylon sutures were used. Dr Saini beautifully cut the diseased cornea and replaced it with the donor cornea. As he passed the first suture and tied the knot, he asked me to cut the end. This nylon suture was very fine, much thinner than human hair, so it was impossible to see it through the naked eye. This was my first time assisting in a corneal transplantation. I tried to cut the suture while looking through the side tube of the operating microscope. No one had explained to me how to use the operating microscope or adjust the interpupillary distance (IPD). 'Suresh,' Dr Saini said, sharply, 'Do not move your scissors in the air. You are just guessing while cutting the suture.' I was taken aback. 'You need to check your refraction tomorrow and ensure that you have 100 per cent precision, not 1 per cent guesswork.' I couldn't respond to Dr Saini, I stood there, stock-still.

But Dr Saini was a kind man. After completing the surgery, he told me the five qualities of an expert surgeon—a lady's fingers, which meant gentle handling; a lion's heart or boldness in decision-making and prompt action; an eagle's eye or watchfulness; a horse's legs, which meant exceptional stamina to stand for hours on end, if needed; and a camel's belly or the ability to carry out work without food and water. Then Dr Saini emphasized on the vision. 'If anyone lacks stereopsis (binocular 3D vision),' he said, 'it would be better for that person to become a non-operating ophthalmologist.' I didn't have it. Despite his explanation, Dr Saini's words felt like a crushing blow. But I did what I always did: I carried on.

## Dr X is Delicate; Dr Y's Hands are Like a Hammer

Throughout my training, I heard a lot about the importance of having a 'surgical hand' in the operating room. If nurses spoke about doctors, they mostly said, 'Dr X is a fine surgeon whose hands are delicate and suitable for microsurgery'. Or 'Dr Y is a bad surgeon and his hands are like a hammer and not at all suitable for eye microsurgery'. When I would hear comments like these, I would look down at my own fingers and hands. Was I even suitable for ophthalmology? I would also get a few seniors to inspect the quality of my hands.

I was worried that if I turned out to be an incompetent surgeon, I would be forced to continue with medical ophthalmology. During this time, my senior, Dr Sangeet Mittal, reassured me. 'Suresh,' he said, 'this is normal. No one explained to you how to use the side tube of the operating microscope. How would you have known?' he asked. 'You should first adjust the interpupillary distance and then use both your eyes to appreciate the depth perception.' He encouraged me to first focus on earning my degree. 'Do you know the golden rule of the medical profession?' he asked. 'Rule number one: the boss is always right; and rule number two, when the boss is wrong, refer to rule number one.' He advised me to be courteous and polite, or risk losing not only a chance to perform surgery but also my degree. I nodded and decided to do as I was told. It wasn't so much the degree that worried me; I didn't want to lose a chance to hone my surgical skills.

## How I Honed My Surgical Skills

Despite the assistance, I didn't get a chance to hone my surgical skills till I reached the USA. There, every weekend, I practised surgery on postmortem eyes in the experimental lab of Professor David Apple's centre. These skills were later enhanced in Australia. I remember doing my first case of phacoemulsification in topical anesthesia at Westmead Hospital in Sydney under Dr Anthony J. Maloof's supervision. Dr Maloof took ten minutes, while I took almost forty-five. The patient heard the conversation as Dr Maloof taught and guided me at each step. But when the surgery was completed and I opened the drapes, I was faced with the patient's wrath. 'Doctor, why did you take almost one hour?' he said. 'You do not know how to operate? You learned on my eyes? Don't learn from the eyes of other patients in Australia. You are a very bad and lousy surgeon and would never become a fast surgeon like Dr Maloof.'

I was humiliated. My eyes welled up and I averted my gaze. Slowly, it started dawning upon me that perhaps I would never become a competent eye surgeon. Later, once I had changed out of my scrubs, Dr Maloof comforted me. 'Never ever be discouraged by such incidents,' he said. He reminded me that Sydney Eye Hospital and Westmead Hospitals were teaching hospitals. The cataract IOL surgery is done free of cost for all patients there as almost every surgery is done by the residents and fellows. The patient, as all patients are, was told in advance that the registrars/fellows would be doing the cataract surgery. If they were not okay with it, they could have gone to a private clinic. 'Every one of us has gone through such tough phases in life. You should take it as a challenge and promise yourself that you would prove him wrong and become one of the best eye surgeons in the world.'

His words of encouragement helped me overcome the crushing sadness I had felt. I kept recalling them for many days to feel better. Once again, I returned to the wet lab. Dr Maloof explained my mistakes to me. He also told me that once I performed surgeries on more eyes, my speed would improve. Performing phaco surgery is like flying an airplane or driving a car, he explained. The more you practice, the better you get. Encouraged by his suggestion, I made it my life's mission to become the best eye surgeon. I wrote it in my diary and stuck a handwritten note on the wall: Dr Suresh

K. Pandey, best eye surgeon. I read it every day to remind myself to move forward toward my dream of becoming one of the best eye surgeons in the world.

Along the way, many surgeons assisted me in my efforts. Dr E. John Milverton, one of my mentors at Sydney Eye Hospital, suggested that I record each surgery and watch the video to catch my mistakes and learn. I acted upon his advice and began to record videos of all my surgeries. With persistence, perseverance and constant positive affirmation, my surgical skills gradually started improving. I also made it a point to pause and reflect on what I had achieved. As author Gaur Gopal Das writes in his book, *Life's Amazing Secrets*, 'Stop and reflect on your life regularly. Pressing the pause button to practice gratitude is the way to make it a constant in your life'.

One day, I noticed that Dr Milverton was going to perform cataract surgery of the right eye with his right hand and the left eye with his left. I was confused. On another day, while imparting pearls of surgical wisdom, Dr Milverton drew something using his left hand. I asked him how he learned to draw with his left hand. 'I was left-handed as a child,' Dr Milverton said. 'I was forced to become right-handed by my teachers. They would often hit my left hand with a cane to stop me from using it. But it is still active.'

I was left-handed and asked Dr Milverton how I too could learn to use both hands and become an ambidextrous surgeon. Dr Milverton suggested that I start training my right hand—using it to brush my teeth and drawing triangles and circles. Now the tough part was to find the time for practising with my non-dominant hand. Every Wednesday and Friday, I would take a train to Westmead Hospital. The journey would take forty-five minutes. I began to utilize this time to draw circles and triangles, and write my name. Within a month, I started doing a few steps of surgery using my right hand, thus taking my first steps on the path to becoming an ambidextrous eye surgeon. But my skills didn't improve overnight.

I spent two years in Australia and performed close to 1,200 minor and major eye surgeries, including cataract surgery (phacoemulsification), pterygium, LASIK laser refractive surgery, corneal transplantation and others. I soon became confident in my cataract surgery skills in both routine and difficult cases. Perhaps I was ready to come to India, but more importantly, I was ready to impart my skills to other unconfident doctors like me, who never thought they would make it.

* * *

While everybody knows it is impossible to truly become ambidextrous, you can get to the point where you can do things with your non-dominant hand. I am naturally left-handed but through practice, I am now able to write with my right hand, use it for surgery and do many other tasks. It is imperative to practise daily. I was practising while commuting from Sydney to Westmead (Australia) each Wednesday and Friday.

Here are a few suggestions to aid new surgeons in training their non-dominant hand:

- Write at least one page daily with your non-dominant hand. You can start with five to ten lines and slowly increase the limit. Try to write numbers.
- Along with writing, also try to draw basic shapes: square, circle, straight lines, etc.
- Perform some daily tasks such as brushing your teeth, eating with a spoon, controlling the mouse while using the PC or using the mobile with the non-dominant hand.
- Write with your non-dominant hand in air.
- Do more and more tasks with your non-dominant hand such as eating, cutting vegetables, etc. to improve precision.

## Lessons Learned after One Lakh Eye Surgeries

Many residents and visiting doctors asked me what the qualities of a good surgeon are. How can they minimize errors and achieve nearly perfect outcomes after each and every surgery?

A good surgeon is one who is attentive, analytical, and eager to learn. The surgeon and team must follow all protocols and the WHO (World Health Organization) checklist to minimize errors such as surgery on the wrong site. When in doubt, a good surgeon never hesitates to take a second opinion. The surgeon must train his entire team to check and cross-check each and every minute detail to avoid any error.

Avoid operating when you are tired. Always have a good night's sleep and prepare your team to deliver the best outcomes. Professor Frank Billson would always emphasize, 'Good surgeons know how to operate, better ones when to operate, and the best when not to operate.' This famous saying surely applies to all fields of medicine. It takes wisdom, experience, strength and courage not to surgically intervene. The minute that a surgeon cuts the skin or a physician prescribes a drug, harm is done. He would direct us to an article titled 'Knowing When Not to Operate',* published in the *British Medical Journal*.

The benefit of a treatment will have to outlast and outdo the harm before a doctor can be said to be doing good. Unfortunately, many treatments have no benefit or only marginal benefit.

---

* 'Knowing when not to operate', *BMJ*, 1999, p. 318.

# 18

# Shaping the Future

## The Power of Mentorship

*'If I didn't have mentors, I wouldn't be here today.'*

—Indra Nooyi

I was always fond of teaching. As a senior medical student, I would often help my juniors with their coursework. In 1993, I appeared in the pre-PG examination and secured the seventh rank. This was the first time Pre-PG started and MBBS graduates appeared for the examination to get admission into postgraduation degree courses. While pursuing ophthalmology in Jabalpur in 1994, I took several classes, conducted rapid-fire sessions as well as mock examinations for young doctors preparing for the Pre-PG examination. I also contributed chapters and MCQs in the several Pre-PG books written by Dr M.S. Bhatia.

During 1998–2005, I continued to share what I knew with colleagues in the USA and Australia, but when I returned to India, I took a plunge into entrepreneurship. Suddenly, I had no time. I was so busy managing my practice that I had almost no time to read, study, or participate in any conferences. I kept feeling like I was missing something important, something close to my heart. When I sat by myself and reflected, the answer came to me. I missed being able to share knowledge with my colleagues to help them. I decided I needed to act upon this desire. I had to find a different way to share my knowledge if travelling or attending conferences was becoming impossible with a young enterprise. The answer came to me, eventually: a YouTube channel. By now, our channel has more than 350 videos with a total viewership of more than 250,000. Slowly, my surgical videos were being watched by eye surgeons worldwide.

I was working in the USA when I first heard about YouTube. I also came across interesting videos related to eye surgery. In 2010, I created my YouTube Channel and uploaded my first video on Toric intraocular lens (IOL) implantation. More than 11,000 eye surgeons saw this video where I shared secrets of Toric IOL implantation. The toric lens were newly introduced in India during that time and used for patients undergoing cataract surgery with corneal astigmatism. We have also submitted these educational videos to the American Academy of Ophthalmology, the American Society of Cataract and Refractive Surgery, and EyeTube, where it became the Editors' Choice. These educational videos were seen and appreciated by the ophthalmology residents, fellows and colleagues worldwide.

After the terrific response to the first video, I was hooked. Dr Vidushi and I began to record many more videos and the response was completely unexpected. Shortly after launching our YouTube Channel, I received an email from Dr Mubariz Qaharmanov from Azerbaijan. He asked if he could come to Kota to observe Dr Vidushi and me while performing surgery. I had never hosted a doctor before, but the more I thought about the email, the more I felt encouraged to do so. I sent Dr Qaharmanova a confirmation and he became the first non-Indian doctor to visit us in Kota. Dr Qaharmanov had completed his ophthalmology training from the National Institute of Ophthalmic Science, Bako, Azerbaijan. But he lacked surgical exposure. I received an excited and enthused Dr Qaharmanov at Kota station and tackled the many questions on his mind.

'Dr Pandey,' he said, 'I have been following you on social media for the past three years. I am so impressed with your journey and with the fact that you started from scratch. The great thing I found about you and Dr Vidushi is that you always share your success so you can help young ophthalmic surgeons start their own journey. Can you please share the secrets of your successful practice with me?'

I learned from Dr Qaharmanov that most doctors prefer visiting a model of eye care delivery that they can reproduce. Many visit renowned institutes and universities to absorb their best practices. But they also realize, in the process, that it is almost impossible to reproduce it. How to navigate medical/ophthalmic entrepreneurship is not a subject taught through any medical curriculum. It has to be figured out the hard way. As Dr Qaharmanov asked his questions, I realized that this was a major contribution I could make to the world of ophthalmology. I could share my story with the world and help those who wanted to learn about a compact, economical and efficient model of delivering eye care services.

Dr Qaharmanov wanted to set up a private ophthalmic practice and I could help him do that. But first, he had to brush up on his surgical skills. He was interested in learning the art of oculoplastic and ophthalmic microsurgery. He was also keen to observe the model of high-volume eye surgery wherein all kinds of eye surgeries are done economically, with utmost efficiency, by employing a caring and compassionate bedside etiquette. And then, when the time was ripe, he could learn the ropes of entrepreneurship: how to start a practice; how to build a team; how to build a patient base, etc.

First, Dr Qaharmanov watched us perform LASIK laser refractive surgery, topical phacoemulsification and multifocal/ toric IOL implantation, suture-less, glue-free, pterygium surgery, strabismus surgery, and many others. He then assisted Dr Vidushi in performing various types of oculoplastic surgery. After thorough and exhaustive surgical exposure, I shared with him my A–F of running a successful practice: A for Availability; B for Behaviour; C for Care, Competence, Compassion; D for Delivery (of the best possible services); E for Exceeding patient's expectations; and F for Feedback (from patients to improve services). Dr Qaharmanov saw how all routine OPD and operated cases were telephoned periodically to enquire about their eye condition and were provided the best possible consultation experience, even if they were away from the city.

Dr Qaharmanov's visit from Azerbaijan caught the fancy of the local press and was also held as a testament to the rising influence of the internet and social media. How the world could descend in a place that doesn't even have a functional airport. Today, Dr Qaharmanov has established his own ophthalmic practice and is doing exceedingly well. He gets in touch with me and fondly remembers the early surgical and entrepreneurial lessons that serve as the compass for his practice today.

## Karachi Calling

As I continued sharing videos of difficult cases on YouTube, EyeTube, Facebook and other social media platforms, I started receiving several invitations to participate in conferences and perform live surgeries. In 2016, I received an invitation from Professor Tariq Aziz of the South Asian Association for Regional Cooperation (SAARC) Academy of Ophthalmology held at Karachi, Pakistan, from 18–21 August 2006.

My visit to Karachi was different from my visit to other countries. Firstly, I received the visa only seventy-two hours before travel. Initially, fourteen eye surgeons were planning to participate in this conference but ten ophthalmologists cancelled their plan at the last minute due to security concerns. I boarded an Emirates flight on 18 August 2006 and reached Karachi (via Dubai), together with four Indian ophthalmologists—Dr Abhay R. Vavavada, Late Dr

V. Sambasiva Rao, Dr Dinesh Talwar and Dr Pukhraj Rishi. We received a grand welcome from the Pakistani ophthalmologists. It was one of the most memorable visits for me and my colleagues, despite our families' concerns about our security there.

I very much enjoyed the SAARC conference—a unique opportunity to meet and interact with Pakistani ophthalmologists. A few of them were Hindus, who had stayed on in Pakistan during the Partition. When it was my turn to speak, Professor Salim Mahar introduced me to the audience. 'I watched Dr Pandey's video on YouTube,' he said. 'It is very difficult to perform phacoemulsification surgery in a sitting position, but Dr Pandey did it. From today, I will call Dr Pandey, Dr Panga.' The audience burst into laughter and then clapped for Professor Mahar.

Our own exchange programme also continued. If I wasn't attending conferences myself, doctors from all over the world would write to me and ask to visit Kota. And all of this because I had started religiously uploading videos on YouTube. It was incredible. By 2019, more than 100 eye surgeons from Azerbaijan, Saudi Arabia, Iraq, Ireland as well as across India, have visited Kota to get advanced training in eye microsurgery. They were not just interested in honing their skills, but also understanding how Dr Vidushi and I ran our hospital.

Dr Qaharmanov's short stint with us not only helped transform his career but also helped us expand our practice. Dr Vidushi launched www.phacolasiktraining.com, a website to help surgeons visit Kota for surgical training. We also continued posting educational videos on YouTube, EyeTube, ophthalmic social media platforms, etc. and many surgeons would arrive to observe our efficiently run private eye hospital setup in a non-metro city, without frills, where you could still get good services.

We also became the first centre in Rajasthan to acquire the Kitaro's dry and wet lab kits. Invented in Japan, the Kitaro kits are an innovative training tool for eye surgeons that allow them to practise cataract surgery using artificial nuclei and lenses. It was Dr Vidushi's brainchild, who firmly believes that all small-incision cataract surgery steps, complication management and common mistakes, use of phacoemulsification equipment, surgical microscope, hand–eye coordination, etc., can be mastered through repeated practice with this revolutionary learning tool. So far, more than sixty ophthalmologists from around the world have trained in phacoemulsification using Kitaro's dry and wet lab training kit at SuVi Eye Institute Kota. While nothing can replace a real human eye, the system is a good adjunct to start surgical training.

One day, I received an email from Dr Linda Vargas, an eye surgeon from Austin, Texas, USA enquiring about visiting Kota for advanced training. I rechecked her qualifications. I was surprised that a surgeon from the USA was keen to visit Kota and learn from us. Dr Vargas had watched several of our surgical videos of routine and complex eye surgeries and was highly impressed by our surgical skills. She was aware that we offered high-quality eye care that involved all types of routine and complex ophthalmic surgeries as well as free eye surgeries to needy patients. But the real reason for Dr Vargas's visit was rooted in her own sense of purpose. She was committed to her job and had conducted many trips to developing countries. But one thing frustrated her on all those journeys: trying to perform intensive surgeries on a dense cataract. She wanted to learn how to perform Small-Incision Cataract Surgery (SICS) and also to fine-tune her skills for performing complex phacoemulsification surgery. SICS is used heavily in the developing world to perform high-volume cataract surgery. This technique is not machine-dependent and is highly affordable in comparison to phacoemulsification. She had watched our videos where we performed SICS, and was eager to come to Kota and learn for herself. Dr Vargas's surgical confidence was also compromised due to a gap in her career. But once she was in Kota, she observed and practised and was able to fine-tune her surgical skills.

Since then, she has helped several thousand people affected by cataracts in the developing world. Her visits as a volunteer eye surgeon in conjunction with several non-profit organizations—such as Orbis International, Sight Savers International, SEE International, Himalayan Cataract Project, Vision Health International—have not only created tremendous impact, but also inspired many to follow in her footsteps. That the training she received at our hospital has strengthened her sight-restoring work from Nepal to Ethiopia, Ghana, and Cuba, makes me feel proud every single day. It reminds me of what Oprah Winfrey said about mentorship, 'A mentor is someone who allows you to see the hope inside yourself'.

# 19

# Blurring Borders

## Treating Patients from Around the World

*'Humanity is an ocean; if a few drops of the ocean are dirty, the ocean does not become dirty.'*

—Mahatma Gandhi

Many Indian parents discourage their children from showing off their achievements. My family was no different. But the more I explored how the world works, the more I moved away from this advice. I realized that marketing hesitation is unproductive; it is at loggerheads with our current world that prioritizes self-promotion and brand-building. I was already absorbed in patient care, but I also wanted to add teaching and training to my repertoire. With this aim, I started a YouTube channel and started uploading surgical videos almost every week since 2010. YouTube's reach was better than anything I could ever have imagined. People from all over the world were watching our videos. We acquired close to 15,000 subscribers and hundreds of queries about our services. YouTube didn't just help bring ophthalmologists from around the world to India, it also helped blur geographical boundaries and bring patients.

## From Kurdistan to Kota

Dr Saman Akram, an eye surgeon from Kurdistan, Iraq paid us a visit, once. Dr Akram's story continues to move me to this day. He was born in 1984, in a Kurdish village, at the time of the Anfal genocide, at the peak of the Iran–Iraq war. This conflict did not leave the Akram family untouched. Dr Akram's father and several male family members went missing. That's when his mother decided to take young Saman and flee. They left their village to live in a suburb of Baghdad. His mother had seen the suffering, the hatred, the loss of life, and wanted revenge. But she decided that her son would become a healer, though there was one problem. Saman's eyes were different from the others. There was an abnormal separation between them. His mother took him to an ophthalmologist in Iraq who told her that it was a congenital problem known as blepharophimosis, ptosis, and epicanthus inversus syndrome (BPES). This is a rare developmental condition affecting the eyelids, which means that at the time of birth, four major features are present: narrow eyes, droopy eyelids, an upward fold of skin of the inner lower eyelids, and wide-set eyes. These features pose difficulty in opening the eyes fully and may affect an individual's quality of vision. A condition like this requires corrective surgery, but only a few trained oculoplastic surgeons can do this. Saman was told that it could only be done after he turned eighteen.

So Saman and his mother learnt to live with it. But Saman's classmates could not. His eyes looked half-opened and gave the impression of sleepiness or inattentiveness. His classmates latched on to this feature of his appearance and began to bully him. Teachers, too, scolded him for being inattentive in class. They didn't understand that he had a rare eye disorder and the young boy had to always keep his chin raised to see properly. Every day, Saman would return home crying, because of all the ridicule, and his mother would console him and promise him that an angel from heaven would fix his eyes through His feather touch. This is how their days passed.

Saman studied long and hard under his mother's care and guidance, who supported the house by running a small grocery store. Saman slowly learnt to ignore his classmates and focus on his education. When he was in standard five, he topped his class and came home and announced that he wanted to become an eye doctor. His mother was ecstatic. To prepare for the medical college entrance examination, Saman was enrolled in a coaching class but had to drop out when his mother was unable to afford the fee. As it turned out, he didn't need coaching.

July 2002 was a great time in the life of eighteen-year-old Saman Akram. He was admitted to the medical college at Al-Mustansiriya University, Baghdad. But here, too, the ridicule didn't stop. His classmates and seniors continued to make fun of his eyes. But Saman focused on his degree and later, his internship. After completing his internship at the same university, he discussed with his mother and decided to get some ophthalmology training outside Iraq. His country was war-torn and unstable, and Dr Saman Akram needed a way out. During his internship, he had grown close to Saddam Hussein's personal doctor and had also had the opportunity to visit the palace a few times. Dr Akram had already been learning how the world worked.

After completing his internship, he left to pursue his ophthalmology training in Ukraine. But there, his rare eye condition got more attention than ever. This time, patients asked him, 'Dr Akram, why do you always look sleepy? Are you taking drugs?' 'First, fix your own eyes before you examine mine', said another patient. Saman knew that he had to treat his eyes. He was operated in Ukraine in 2009 but the problem recurred after a few months as the sutures used for the corrective surgery were absorbed. In the meantime, he completed his training. Three years ago, he had become a doctor and realized his mother's dream. But now, it was time to overcome the challenge that had been nagging at him for the past twenty-eight years—his rare eye disorder.

There were not many trained oculoplastic surgeons in Iraq or Ukraine. And surgery in the US or Europe would have proved to be prohibitively expensive. Dr Akram needed a cost-effective solution. One day, while browsing the internet, he came across one of Dr Vidushi's videos. They were on the very condition that he had. Dr Akram could not believe it. He dreamt about flying to India and getting the procedure done. He contacted us through Facebook Messenger and emailed us his case history. We prepared an invitation letter to make it easier for him to get a visa and as soon as the formalities were completed, he was ready to come. At the time, he was working at an eye hospital in Sulemania. He took a flight from Baghdad to Jaipur and then took a train to Kota; he stayed in a guest room at SuVi Eye Hospital.

Dr Akram, Dr Vidushi and I had a chance to talk about his life. He told us about the many ways in which this rare eye condition had affected his self-esteem. Not only during his growing years but also now, as he was struggling to find a suitable life partner. One of his biggest problems was that his patients would often look at him and ask, 'Dr Akram, why do you not treat your own eyes?'

Dr Vidushi examined his eyes carefully and told him that she would conduct the surgery under general anaesthesia. She would use a non-absorbable suture to correct the droopy eyelids. On 24 May 2013, Dr Vidushi performed the sling surgery to improve droopy eyelids. In about 100 minutes, the surgery was completed. There was some swelling on his eyelid, the next day, but the palpebral aperture of his both eyes increased significantly. Dr Akram looked into the mirror and exclaimed, 'Wow! I can't believe it! My prayers have been answered!' He thanked us profusely. But he didn't know that we had another surprise for him. After we heard his story, we decided to not charge him for his surgery.

When he resisted, Dr Vidushi said that she had received the message to perform the surgery from an angel. Dr Akram couldn't hold back his tears. He called his mother and got her to speak to us. His mother struggled to speak but we knew that her happiness knew no bounds. After the successful sling surgery, there was considerable improvement in the palpebral aperture of both his eyes. But that wasn't the end of our engagement. We had in our care, not just a patient but an ophthalmologist from Iraq. We encouraged Dr Akram to attend our surgery sessions. He asked many questions and attended the surgical cases in the operating room. Over the years, I have stayed in touch with him. He is now married and has two beautiful children.

The story of Dr Saman Akram is one of struggle and determination, but also the story of how the world is made of artificial borders that prevent us from being fully human. A few YouTube videos brought him to Kota and reiterated how it's important to not just do good work but to always be willing to learn, experiment and evolve with time. If you want to gain a competitive edge in your profession, you have to stay in sync with the rising trends. It is patients and collaborators like Dr Saman Akram who motivate us to push and work harder. To build institutions and processes synonymous with excellence, whose cornerstones are care, compassion and commitment for people transcending borders.

## Medical Tourism: A Journey From Karachi to Kota

India and Pakistan share a troubled border despite many efforts to establish peace. Many patients, especially children, have come to India from Pakistan to receive medical treatment as well as undergo surgical procedures at bigger hospitals.* However, the story I'm

---

* Ferya Ilyas, 'Medical tourism: In Indian hospitals, life-saving treatments for Pakistani patients', *The Express Tribune Pakistan*. Available at: https://tribune.com.pk/story/1184276/medical-tourism-indian-hospitals-life-saving-treatments-pakistani-patients.

sharing here is that of Fahim Uddin, a software engineer working at the Orthopaedic and Medical Institute, Karachi, Pakistan, who was myopic and had developed cataracts at about forty years of age. His Internet search had led him to IOL websites and he decided he wanted a particular multifocal IOL (Tecnis Multifocal IOL, Johnson and Johnson, USA), which was not available in Pakistan at the time. He then searched for the IOL in India and found many videos that I had posted on the implantation of this IOL. He communicated with us through social media and after a few interactions, developed so much trust in us that he decided to come to India for the surgery.

Fahim arrived on a medical visa and underwent cataract surgery in both eyes with the multifocal IOL of his choice at SuVi Eye Institute in July 2012, and was extremely happy with the results. He even watched a Bollywood movie (*Bol Bachchan*) in the theatres immediately after the surgery and toured the city of Kota, thrilled with the excellent vision he had—both distance and near, without glasses, with no significant night vision problems either.

The fact that he had come over from Karachi for his eye surgery made him something of a mini-celebrity and his visit was well-covered by the local media. A programme, 'Spreading Light Across the Border' (*Aman Ki Roshni*) was organized during his visit and the Mayor of Kota at the time, Dr Ratna Jain, the Inspector General of Police, Shri Amrit Kalash, and some other prominent local personalities also participated in it. His visit to India was a unique case of human trust and empathy that knew no boundaries, neither political nor religious. When it comes to interpersonal interactions, Indians and Pakistanis have always been very warm towards each other, in my experience, and this was just another reinforcement of the need for the two neighbours to live like friends.

When I visited Karachi for the SAARC Conference during 18–21 August 2016, Fahim showed me around the city. He made the trip even more memorable for me.

# 20

# 'Guarda La Luce'

## Looking Towards the Light

*'If you can put a positive affirmation in your mind and can hold on to it, you can make it happen. The longer you hold on to it, the more you dwell upon it, the more are its chances of becoming real.'*

—Ralph Marston

It was 26 October 2005. As I drove to the Sydney International Airport, I was a bag of nerves. It was going to be a twenty-two-hour flight to Milan, Italy. I had a big lump in my throat. I kept wondering what made me agree to this. I was going for a conference as I had many times before, but this was different. I was going to perform a live surgery. Conferences are cradles for surgical as well as research work, and top academics and researchers congregate for these events. My academic credentials and professional networking ensured that I received an invitation to perform live surgery at a very early stage of my surgical career—in fact, during my fellowship training itself. But I was not sure about my ability to do it.

## Getting Inspired by the Inventor of Phacoemulsification

Performing a live surgery during an international conference is a matter of great honour and prestige, and is reserved for the best and the most experienced surgeons alone. Even they get anxious during live surgery, as one's most highly qualified colleagues are watching. And here I was, pretty much a novice. But the more I thought about the invitation, the more I convinced myself to try. So I gave it a shot. I got off the cab and braced myself for a long flight to Italy. My mind flashed images of all the surgeries I had performed so far. Somewhere in the corner, there was also the story of Dr Charles D. Kelman. As I thought about my journey of moving ahead with the phacoemulsification technique, I found many similarities with the technique's inventor—Dr Charles D. Kelman. From 1964 to 1968, Dr Kelman had been hard at work but had nothing to show for it. He was tired, frustrated and badly in need of a dentist.

When he sat in the dentist's chair, something changed. As the dentist Dr Larry Kuhn brought out the ultrasonic scaler to clean his teeth, Dr Kelman got an idea. He could use the ultrasonic phaco technology to emulsify the cataract. And just like that, he had cracked it. I didn't have an invention to my name, but like Dr Kelman, after years of struggling to improve my surgical skills, I had crushed the block and become a competent and confident surgeon. And now, I was going to Milan to demonstrate my surgical prowess—live.

## The Challenge of the First Live Surgery and Chairman's Advice

I was nervous but it was for good reason. At Milan, I had to perform live surgery on an Alcon Infiniti phaco machine, which had been recently launched by Alcon Surgical, USA. But there was no Infiniti machine at the time, at Sydney Eye Hospital. I wasn't sure if I could pull off a live surgery on a machine I wasn't even familiar with. Ten days before Milan, I was due to attend another conference by the American Academy of Ophthalmology in Chicago. Here, I asked Professor Randall J. Olson (Chairman, John A. Moran Eye Centre, University of Utah, Salt Lake City, USA) whether I should accept the invitation to Milan. 'I would not accept this invitation,' Professor Olson said. 'What if something went wrong with this new machine? It would spoil your inner confidence.' Professor Olson was right—he also suggested that I could request them to make the machine I was familiar with, available. But by then I had conjured up an entirely new idea.

Through the corner of my eye, I spied that the new Infiniti® phaco machine was on display at the conference in Chicago. This was my opportunity. I talked to representatives of the company and asked if I could practise and familiarise myself with the machine. It is not uncommon for experienced surgeons to perform surgeries on new models of phaco machines during conferences. But this was my first time and I did not want to take any chances, especially when a human eye was involved. I practised performing a few surgeries using model eyes during the AAO Conference in Chicago and then ten days later, I was in Milan.

It was a crisp October morning in Milan when I landed after a long flight, and I was exhausted. The organizer, Professor Lucio Buratto's team, arrived to receive me at the airport and take me to the Hilton where I was staying. Very soon, I would have to demonstrate my skills in front of 1,500 eye surgeons during the live surgery program on 28 October 2005.

## Guarda La Luce: Look to the Light

It was the morning of 28 October 2005. It was going to be one of the most important days of my life. I had learnt the art of microsurgery and now I had to demonstrate it. But there was also doubt. Despite my efforts to rouse my confidence, I also recalled instances when both doctors and patients had expressed doubt in my abilities. Yet, here I was. The live surgery event was organized at the Centro Ambrosiano di Microchirurgia Oculare (or CAMO, now known as the clinic Centro Ambrosiano Oftalmico)—one of the most famous eye institutes in Milan. Before me, the most renowned surgeons had been invited to participate in the live surgery event. But today was my turn and I was determined to do well.

I entered the operation theatre, nervous and stressed. Dr Lucio Buratto had introduced me. I greeted the audience of 1,500 eye surgeons from around the world by saying '*Buongiorno*' or 'good morning' in Italian. 'I am Dr Suresh K. Pandey,' I said. 'I come from Australia and I am here to demonstrate to you my technique of phacoemulsification and implantation of Alcon AcrySof Restor intraocular lens.' I was nervous and wasn't sure if my voice exuded confidence, but I reassured myself that everything would go well. The audiovisual team fitted a mic on my body. I adjusted the eyepiece of the operating microscope, the height of the operating table, and checked the footswitch of the operating microscope and phaco machine. I then positioned the patient's chin and eye so that I could demonstrate the live surgery efficiently.

I was worried about the entire surgery—all its steps, as well as other major details, such as conducting the surgery on topical anaesthesia in a non-English-speaking country. When the surgeon performs cataract surgery using topical anaesthesia, it is important for the patient's eye to fixate on the light of the operating microscope. This often means telling the patient to look towards the light. I could comfortably do this in Australia but how would I do it in Milan? I found a simple solution of learning how to say the phrase in Latin: 'Guarda la luce,' I told my patient during the live surgery. I began the surgery by creating a side port incision. Then, I injected the viscoelastic, a jelly-like substance into the eye to create a space and protect the delicate endothelial cells. After that, I created a capsulorhexis, 5 mm in size. I emulsified Grade 3 hard cataract using an ultrasonic needle connected to the Alcon Infiniti phacoemulsification machine. This was followed by the removal of cortical matter by bimanual irrigation and aspiration. I filled the capsular bag with viscoelastic and implanted AcrySof Restor IOL in the capsular bag using the Monarch Injector. The surgery was over within thirteen minutes. The hall erupted into applause and I looked up, finally relieved.

'Thank you, Dr Pandey, for your demonstration of the surgery done very elegantly,' Professor Lucio Buratto said. I was suddenly showered with appreciation and congratulations as I was perhaps one of the youngest surgeons to perform live surgery before an audience of world-renowned doctors.

## Talk While You Perform Surgery

I wasn't going to leave Milan after merely demonstrating my abilities and learning nothing. In fact, I learnt a very important lesson from George Briscoe. George was an employee of Alcon Surgical and had excellent knowledge of the Alcon Infiniti Machine. When I met him, I was happy and relieved that I could ask him about the machine setting. He was a big help to me. He also gave me another important message. 'I have been assisting various eye surgeons on the phaco machine for the past thirty years,' he said. 'And, there's only one thing you should know: always talk to your patients while performing surgery. Make this an important habit and this would make the patient comfortable and also you would never have any stress or anxiety while performing live surgery.'

It was simple advice but its effect was truly phenomenal. I put this advice in practice as soon as I returned to Australia and it really did wonders for my confidence and precision. But I felt its true impact in India. One day, an elderly woman came to me for cataract treatment. While operating on her, I asked her about her family members to start a conversation and keep her distracted from the fear of surgery. The lady sounded very disturbed while talking about her son. She told me about his alcoholism and how he had lost his family due to his addiction. I refrained from asking further but she volunteered more information—how he was a genius before addiction gripped him; how he knew five languages and had an excellent job. But alas, everything was destroyed. I felt a deep pang of sadness upon hearing this. I reassured her that I would visit her house and counsel her son. But after two days, she visited the hospital herself with her son, who was now developing an eye problem.

After completing his examination and giving him medications, I took the son aside and told him how his mother was in tears when I asked her about him. 'Your mother is proud of you and she told me you can speak five languages. You were a genius before you developed this addiction,' I said and shortly after, forgot all about the incident. A few months later, the mother and son visited me again. The mother was beaming—he had quit drinking. I couldn't believe my ears. I wondered what had happened—was it the fact that the advice had come from a doctor? The son later confided that when I talked to him about his problems in a kind and compassionate manner, he felt ashamed that a doctor they visit probably once a year could feel his mother's pain, and not him. This pricked his conscience.

But it wasn't just his own life that changed. He worked with me to help many alcoholic patients give up drinking. Unfortunately, he passed away in 2020. I was deeply gratified that my advice had changed someone's life. I silently thanked George. Today, in 2023, I have successfully performed 1 lakh phacoemulsification and intraocular lens implantation surgeries. And in most cases, I have also had deep, meaningful conversations with my patients—both before and after the surgery.

## Applying Milan's Live Surgery Lessons in Kota

George Biscoe had the opportunity to visit India in June 2018. He was very happy to come to Kota and spend one day with me in the OT. George told me that while he shared his secret of talking while performing surgery with thousands of eye surgeons in the past, only I had followed his advice sincerely. In Kota, he saw me do it all day as I performed twenty-five cataract surgeries, one after the other.

My staff members, too, follow George Biscoe's million-dollar advice. While I perform surgery in the operating room, the video is telecast live in the waiting room while my staff members add their voiceovers. They begin with the invention of the IOL by Dr Harold Ridley and the invention of phacoemulsification by Dr Charles Kelman, and answer any questions people may have. Sometimes, this is also accompanied by a livestream on social media. During the livestream, we explain each procedure, and answer every question, not just to demonstrate our own skills but to foster and maintain the trust of our patients. By showing every step live on the screen, the patients' worries are better managed and they feel more reassured of the ethos of our work.

# 21

# Interacting with Kota's Coaching Students

*'So often you find that the students you're trying to inspire are the ones that end up inspiring you.'*

—Sean Junkins

In May–June 2017, *Dainik Bhaskar* Kota organized a 'Live Positive Campaign' to spread positivity and happiness among the coaching students of Kota city. Dr Vidushi and I were invited to deliver a series of motivational talks at Kota's famous coaching centres such as Allen Career Institute, Aakash Institute, Resonance Eduventures, Motion Education, Career Point, Sarvottam Career Institute, Nucleus education, Btrix medical classes, etc. Our first lecture was at Sarvottam Career Institute, a coaching institute exclusively for The National Eligibility cum Entrance Test (NEET) (medical) aspirants. When we entered the institute, we were welcomed by the enthusiastic aspirants themselves. One of the faculty members introduced Dr Vidushi and me to a rapt audience. They clapped when they heard that Dr Vidushi completed her MBBS and postgraduate education from AIIMS, New Delhi, and I did my postgraduation from the PGIMER, Chandigarh.

Truth be told, I wanted to clap for them for the role *they* had played in *my* life. When we moved to Kota in December 2005, we never realized that we would meet so many students each and every day. Kota is home to about 2 lakh students, who are mainly NEET and IIT-JEE aspirants. The city never sleeps and there is hustle-bustle around the clock. These students, who visited us for eye check-ups, also became our brand ambassadors, who told others about our services. Many of them visited their grandparents for consultation for cataract or other eye surgery. As I thought about my gratitude for the students, I spared a moment's thought for the man who started it all.

## Beacon of Light: The Story of Mr Vinod Kumar Bansal

On 25 March 2006, a patient came to consult me. Smt. Aruna Gupta was fifty-eight years old and suffering from age-related macular degeneration (ARMD). She underwent multiple anti-vascular endothelial growth factor (VEGF) injections in the left eye while staying with her son in the USA. I examined her retina and performed a fundus fluorescein angiography (FFA) test to evaluate the condition of the retina. The FFA test confirmed the presence of a wet form of ARMD. I took her to the OT to inject an intravitreal injection of Lucentis. Lucentis (ranibizumab) injection is a monoclonal antibody that works by slowing the growth of abnormal new blood vessels in the eye and decreasing leakage from these blood vessels, used to treat the wet form of age-related macular degeneration.

After she was shifted to the operating room (OR), I started talking to her to allay her anxiety. I asked her when she came to India and how she came to know about us. She told me she is the sister of Vinod Kumar Bansal's wife. I told her I heard a lot about Bansal sir, a renowned educationist and the founder of Bansal Classes, a well-known chain of coaching centres and that I really wanted to meet him. I injected the anti-VEGF injection, finished the surgeries for the day and forgot all about the episode. On March 26, I received a call from Mr Bansal. He said, 'Dr Pandey, V.K. Bansal this side. You expressed a desire to meet me. Please come and let us have breakfast together.'

It was a pleasant surprise for me although I could not join him on the day he invited me. I met him a little later, when he arrived for his cataract surgery and lens implantation. The surgery went well and I realized how difficult it was for him to carry out simple everyday tasks, such as wearing and taking off his spectacles, due to his muscular dystrophy. He shared his own story of studying under the lantern and I recalled my own journey of having done the same. But I looked at the man and felt nothing but awe: he had laid the foundation for what Kota is today. All the coaching institutes can be traced back to this great gentleman's pioneering initiative. Like Mr Bansal, there were many students in Kota who left an indelible mark on me.

## Tuhin Dey: The Stephen Hawking of India

On 11 June 2018, I received a phone call from Shri Rajesh Maheshwari, director of Allen Career Institute, to examine the eye of his special student. The student's name was Tuhin Dey. Affected by arthrogryposis multiplex congenita (AMC), a condition that causes joints to be stiff and crooked at birth, he was wheelchair-bound. But the wheelchair didn't dampen his will one bit. He would hold a pen with his mouth to write, and aspired to become a physicist like his world-renowned idol, Stephen Hawking.

As I examined his eyes and checked the power of glasses, all staff members and patients gathered to see this special child. His parents shared his journey. Tuhin had appeared for the CBSE exam from Central School, IIT-Kharagpur in West Midnapore district, West Bengal. He had shifted to Kota a couple of months ago to prepare for the JEE. Seventeen-year-old Tuhin had inched a little closer to his dream as he cleared his CBSE Class 10 examination, scoring 88 per cent.

But going to school and appearing for the Class 10 examination was not easy for Tuhin, who was 90 per cent disabled. However, this never deterred him from his dream of studying in the country's top college. The Kharagpur boy's journey was not easy as he was dependent on others for his daily needs and routine. But the determined Tuhin used his mouth to hold a pen and his chin to operate gadgets like smartphones, tablets and laptops for online learning. In 2020, Tuhin cracked the JEE examination in the general PWD category securing 438th rank. Tuhin's story not only motivated me but also the entire staff of the SuVi Eye Hospital as well as all the patients who had been present on that special day. We learnt from him the power of determination, dedication and sheer willpower to achieve success. I am of the view that the power of the subconscious mind and a sound mental frame is very important to get the desired results from one's life.

## Orphan to Cardiac Surgeon

In February 2006, when we started our practice, we met Akshaya Lohar, a student who came from a Rajgarh village, near Indore. Gadia Lohars (also known as Gaduliya Lohars or Rajput Lohar) are a nomadic community of Rajasthan and the Malwa region of MP. Most of this nomadic community works by the roadside and earns daily wages. Unfortunately, Akshaya lost both of his parents in a road accident. In the tragic accident, Akshaya too was injured badly and suffered multiple bone fractures, but was saved after multiple operations and prolonged treatment at a hospital in Indore. He was shifted to an orphanage, where he continued to excel at his studies. He was committed to becoming a doctor and working as a healer for the rest of his life.

One of the coaching institutes of Kota invited him to study in Kota and promised to bear all his expenses. Akshaya visited SuVi

Eye Hospital for his eye check-up. When we met Akshaya and heard his story, we were in tears. I wrote on his prescription: 'Dr Akshaya, future surgeon'. Recently, we got a message from Dr Akshaya Lohar mentioning that he had completed his MS (Surgery) and was doing a super specialization (MCh) in cardiothoracic and vascular surgery. His story is one of determination, resilience and relentlessness, even during the most adverse situation.

## The Inspiring Story of an Engineering Aspirant

Vikram Shukla had poor vision since childhood due to congenital cataracts in both eyes. He underwent cataract surgery and artificial lens implantation in the left eye at the age of six, in Bhopal, MP. Unfortunately, his vision did not improve significantly. In addition to poor vision, he suffered from pain and redness in his left eye after surgery due to corneal decompensation. He was scared to lose his other eye so, in spite of a very poor vision, he continued to study using his only seeing eye (the right eye).

In 2006, at the age of seventeen, he came to Kota from Guna, MP and joined coaching classes to prepare for the IIT-JEE examination. He consulted me and shared his story in detail. He also told me that he was determined to get selected despite his poor vision and would undergo cataract surgery only after his selection. Vikram mentioned that his elder sister was helping him a lot with his studies. Every day, she would read the text aloud and he would listen to it. I tried to convince him to get the cataract surgery in his right eye so he could study well, but he was not keen due to his underwhelming experience of surgery in the past.

He told me about the way he studied and I was in awe: his sister would read aloud from his books and he would make mental notes. Or he would hold the book very close to his eye and use a magnifying glass to read the text using a bright light. When the IIT-JEE exam came closer, he, his sister and all his family members worked very hard. Finally, their efforts paid off, and he was selected to attend IIT Mumbai. Before joining IIT Mumbai, he came to me and I congratulated him for his great success. He agreed to undergo cataract surgery and lens implantation in the right eye. He asked me to promise him that I would do my best to treat his working eye.

After a comprehensive evaluation, and a detailed check-up, I took up his case. A toric intra-ocular lens (IOL) was selected to address the problem of corneal astigmatism. I performed micro-incision cataract surgery and toric IOL implantation in his right eye. The surgery was successful and he regained 100 per cent vision for near and distance (with glasses). Vikram is now working as an engineer at Bhabha Atomic Research Centre (BARC) Mumbai. Vikram's story taught me that nothing is impossible in life for a determined person. I also learnt how important it is to not lose hope, even in the most adverse situations.

Students like Tuhin, Akshaya and Vikram have taught me more about life than any medical book could've. And I use their example while talking to several other students. But I also remind them that no exam is bigger than that of life, so they must try their hardest and never give up.

## 22

# My Failures, Mistakes and Limitations

## The Importance of Planning Ahead

*'Well begun is half done.'*

—Aristotle

'Papa, why did you return from Sydney?' Ishita once asked me. She sees her parents work extremely hard on a regular basis and often wishes that we had more free time on our hands. While we try our best to balance work and life, sometimes it gets difficult. One day in 2018, we drove from Kota on 14 August to meet Ishita at her boarding school in Jaipur.

Ishita is a creative child, often lost in books, and she had insisted on studying at a boarding school—perhaps to experience a new kind of world that would aid her writing instincts. While we were on our way, the collector of Kota, Gaurav Goyal, IAS, called to inform us that Dr Vidushi had been selected to receive an award on 15 August. Dr Vidushi and I looked at each other and then at Ishita. We didn't want to leave her but we also couldn't disappoint the collector, who had personally called us. It was decided that I would leave for Kota to receive the award on her behalf while Dr Vidushi would stay with

Ishita. It was a tough choice and Ishita was extremely displeased. As was I. On the way, I thought about our decision to return to India.

Staying in India or moving overseas is a personal choice. Both have their pros and cons. When I look back, I realize we not only chose a difficult life over a well-balanced one, but I also hamstrung my professional and personal lives because I was unable to make up my mind about what I wanted to do. Working overseas had several advantages: good starting pay with less frenetic working hours than in India, educated patients, less patient load, more opportunities—you could become a faculty member at a prestigious university (teaching) hospital, publish excellent research papers and keep undergoing medical training. You could also collaborate with world-renowned scientists and experts with far more ease. From a personal standpoint, too, living abroad has its perks in terms of a better quality of life, better lifestyle, facilities and freedom.

But the more time I spent abroad, the more guilty I felt about leaving my country. I was raised and trained in India. How could I reconcile the fact that when the time came to serve my people, I moved away? Some may defend their decision to stay abroad as a personal choice and that's perfectly acceptable, but my conscience kept pricking at me. When I would read about the poor healthcare facilities in India or the frightening doctor–patient ratio, the huge burden of preventable blindness, and the reason for all of it being an extreme dearth of eye doctors, my heart would bleed. Still, I waited and prioritized the honing of my surgical skills. It was not an easy decision to make and I kept putting it off.

Every time I tried to think about returning to India, my mind would be wracked with impossible-to-answer questions: will I get a good enough job? Good salary? Satisfaction? Freedom? The answers were too hard to find and instead of probing further, I would stop thinking about them altogether. The second was a question of finances. Ever since I was a child, I had lacked negotiation skills. I was reticent, unwilling to stick my neck out, and this, I carried with me into my early adulthood. In 2005, after completing my fellowship in Australia, I planned to join a prestigious institute in Hyderabad but was hesitant to discuss the monetary terms. I was also ignorant and assumed that I would be paid handsomely. But when I was told my salary, I was shocked. It was merely a quarter of what I had been expecting. It was also clear to me that important terms have to be discussed upfront. They can't be put off. If, like me, you're not proactive about having these discussions, you would suffer like Dr Vidushi and I did, when we nearly went broke paying our bills.

When Dr Vidushi and I failed to secure good jobs, it was our lack of finances or even financial knowledge that anguished us the most. Here we were, full-grown adults, who didn't understand money. How, then, could we start our own practice? How would we manage patient care and research? If we discussed this with our seniors and friends, they would actively discourage us from going back to India and that often worsened our dilemma. They made us question the kind of environment we would be stepping into. An environment where health was not a priority, but a rather measly proportion of the GDP (1.2 per cent).* At a time when there is such a paucity of doctors across India, there is an increasing saturation of doctors in metro cities. Several new doctors are struggling to earn enough through their newly established clinics. A very limited number of government hospitals offer a liveable salary and good working conditions. Healthcare in India is swarming with challenges. On the one hand, established doctors (or corporate establishments) keep launching new branches, whereas new doctors struggle to make a living. This gap is widening with each passing year in metro cities.

Doctors often meet unique challenges that hinder their financial wellness. These include a lengthy, expensive education, which results

---

* 'India spends just 1.2% of its GDP on healthcare, but a policy can change that', *Business Insider*, 20 June 2018. Available at: https://www.businessinsider.in/india-spends-just-1-2-of-its-gdp-on-healthcare-but-a-policy-can-change-that/articleshow/64665303.cms.

in a mountain of student debt. While most others are well settled in their jobs by their late twenties, doctors are only just getting started and most continue to struggle well into their mid-thirties. How, then, can a doctor plan their finances? Between paying educational loans, setting up a new medical practice and dealing with long erratic working hours, there's little time (or money) to concentrate on learning financial planning. I focused on the negatives and rationalized the decision I was making—I allowed myself to move away from my purpose. Then one day, I attended a conference of the American Society of Cataract and Refractive Surgery (ASCRS) and all my doubts melted away. That day in San Diego, the first Indian doctor, Dr Govindappa Venkataswamy, was being inducted into their Hall of Fame in 2004.

I had met Dr Venkataswamy in 1998 in Madurai when I visited the Aravind Eye Hospital, Madurai. But somehow, in the rush of life, this meeting had been locked away in a corner of my mind vault. The meeting turned out to be the key. Dr Venkataswamy, popularly known as Dr V, was an ophthalmologist who had dedicated his life to eliminating blindness. The founder and former chairman of Aravind Eye Hospitals, he had developed a high-quality, high-volume, low-cost service delivery model that restored the eyesight of millions of people. In the initial years, he and his team faced many financial difficulties. But Dr V founded Seva Foundation (a USA-based non-profit organization), to partner with Aravind in the early years. This expanded the organization's access to the latest technology and skilled volunteers. Seva continues to collaborate with Aravind in various aspects of eye care management, education and research.

I sat there, my skin covered in goosebumps, as I heard that Aravind Eye Care System had examined over 55 million patients and performed over 6.8 million surgeries. And, what was even more remarkable was that over 50 per cent of the organization's patients paid either nothing or highly subsidized rates. Its scale and self-sustainability had prompted a 1993 Harvard Business Case

Study. On the one hand was the system Dr V had set up; on the other was Dr V himself. At thirty, he was permanently crippled by rheumatoid arthritis but had still personally performed over 100,000 eye surgeries. As a government servant, he helped to develop and pioneer the concept of eye camps and received a Padma Shri from the Government of India. Dr V's contribution was unparalleled. In 1992, he and his partners at Aravind founded Aurolab, an internationally certified manufacturing facility, that brought the price of the intraocular lens down to one-tenth of international prices and made it affordable for developing countries.

Today, Aurolab manufactures ophthalmic pharmaceuticals, instruments and equipment, in addition to intraocular lenses, and exports to 160 countries worldwide. In 1996, under Dr Venkataswamy's leadership, the Lions Aravind Institute for Community Ophthalmology (LAICO) was founded. LAICO is a training and consulting institute that has helped replicate the Aravind model in 347 hospitals across India and thirty other developing countries. The knowledge was not brand new, but it was coming to me at a time when I was most receptive to it. It kindled a deep desire in me—a desire to return to my home country and walk in the footsteps of Dr V. To go back to India, where my services were most needed.

Suddenly, there was no dilemma. Dr Vidushi and I decided to put our heads together and achieve entrepreneurial success. We had plenty of resolve but from day one, I was conscious of my limitations. I had trained myself to become a competent eye surgeon, but nothing else. As I struggled to start something new at thirty-eight, I realized how important it is for doctors to understand hospital finances. One should know the basic terminologies and meanings of terms like capital expenses, operational expenses, profit and loss statements, internal rate of return, return on interest and several other terms that used to gobsmack me before. I knew nothing. So if there's one advice I'd love to give young doctors, it's this: take an active interest in financing your life and your profession. And if a good job does come along, don't hesitate to negotiate the salary structure with the management. Many say that it's only those without a plan B who succeed and while it might be true, the stress of not having a backup plan is not always worth it.

Dr Vidushi and I spent the early years of our entrepreneurial career in extreme duress. And almost every other day, I would remember Benjamin Franklin's famous words, 'If you fail to plan, you are planning to fail'. We might have turned the tide, but having well-researched, reviewed and elaborate plans is a far better way of launching any initiative. This is also what will help you manage work and life better—although sacrifices are inevitable. Anything else is a brave folly, as I now realize. Heedless bravery might pay off sometimes, but well-charted and planned efforts almost certainly have a better shot at success.

## 23

# Steel in My Soul

## Daring to Win Big

*'A successful person is one who can lay a firm foundation with the bricks that others throw at him.'*

—David Brinkley

A difficult childhood can propel two kinds of emotions: a breakdown of any ambition or a burning desire for achievement. I felt the latter. I found within myself a strong passion, an internal urge, to become someone significant and do something substantial for society. What reinforced this belief was books. I enjoyed reading and would often raid my father's library as a child. My father had a collection of motivational books by Dr Orison Swett Marden, Shri Ram Sharma Acharya, Ram Charan Mahendra, Osho Rajneesh, Dale Carnegie, Geeta Press Gorakhpur, and many others. It was these books I returned to when I needed to feel energized or hopeful. In 1985–86, when I was preparing for my Pre Medical Test (PMT) to fulfil my dream of becoming an eye doctor, it was a rough time at home. Conflicts were rife and my father's salary barely covered our expenses. I was acutely conscious of the financial crunch and was saving every penny. On one such day, I read a story about Socrates and Plato.

Plato thought Socrates was the wisest person of his time and he passionately desired to learn all of Socrates' wisdom. Legend has it that one day Socrates and Plato were walking down the beach, deep in conversation. At one point, Socrates said to Plato, 'Walk with me into the ocean'. They turned and walked into the sea together. I pictured what was happening. Student and teacher, two of the greatest philosophers, striding into the surf side by side. The water surrounded their ankles, then rose up to their knees. As the water got higher, Plato wondered, 'What is the lesson my master is trying to teach me?' When the water reached the shoulder, Socrates abruptly grabbed Plato's head and pushed him down under the water. Plato, held down, wondered what this lesson was all about. After some time, Plato ran out of air. He began to struggle to get his head above water. He punched and kicked and grabbed in vain to wriggle free, but Socrates was a strong man and held him down. Finally, Plato blacked out due to lack of oxygen. Socrates pulled him ashore and resuscitated him. When Plato regained consciousness, he angrily accused Socrates of trying to drown him. Socrates matter-of-factly explained, 'If that had been my intention, I would not have pulled you ashore.'

'Then why did you do that?' Plato demanded.

Socrates calmly replied, 'When you desire my knowledge like you desired that breath of air, then you shall have it.'

The story invoked many feelings in me. Did I desire passionately enough? Did I really want to become a doctor, achieve financial independence and societal appreciation? And that's when I realized that people who do go after the things they desire, desire them with a wild passion. Such leaders allow and even encourage themselves to desire. They create a hunger within themselves, which pulls them out of their discomfort. I set the book down and nodded. Challenges, adverse circumstances, difficulties—they will come and go. I could not let them disturb my motivation. That night, I wrote a few sentences in my diary: 'I will not feel defeated while overcoming adverse circumstances. My desire to excel will be very intense and I will put 100 per cent effort towards achieving it. I will not play a victim and will not make any excuses. These challenging circumstances are here to make me stronger.' I ended the paragraph with a phrase from author Jan Winebrenner: 'Steel in his soul'. I wrote down that I had steel in my soul.

This is the message I carried with me when I wanted to build a world-class eye institute in India. The excellent training I received in the USA and Australia pushed me to think about the many young doctors who do not get surgical exposure after completing their MS Ophthalmology and then struggle to become competent surgeons. I was also aware of the many challenges in Indian healthcare when it came to effective and affordable treatment. Therefore, I wanted to establish a not-for-profit, non-government, public-spirited, comprehensive academic eye care institution, that could provide ophthalmic training to young eye doctors in North India. And my primary source of inspiration was the many doctors and businesspersons who had established themselves before me.

Initially, I dreamt of setting up a world-class eye hospital and institute in Jaipur. I wrote down my detailed plan of action and an accompanying letter and sent it to India's top fifty businesspersons and doctors. I requested them to give me an appointment so that I could meet them and explain my dream project. Like an institute in Hyderabad received five acres of free land and ₹1 crore in funding, I hoped that I would get at least some funding to fulfil my dream. I emailed the biggest business tycoons of the country and some famous doctors. I did not get any reply from most people. The few who did reply, replied in the negative. I recall a reply from a New York-based eye surgeon who was from Rajasthan and had migrated to the USA. 'It is not possible to establish an eye institute in Rajasthan,' he told me. 'Even if you establish an eye institute by raising money, you cannot run in the long-term as you would not be able to find a capable team. It would be an extremely difficult (almost impossible) job to attract and retain good and capable doctors and staff members. I tried but was not successful.'

His reply crushed me. It took me some time to motivate myself and continue working towards my dream. In December 2005, when Dr Vidushi and I returned to India and started our journey of entrepreneurship, I thought I was on the path to prove him right: I had failed to find funding and instead of a world-class institute, I was starting small with my own funding. But as I remained committed, I realized that I had found a niche for myself: a model of compact ophthalmic practice. It was not only relevant and respected, but also responsible and replicable, even during serious financial crises such as the COVID-19 pandemic.

## International Doctors Visiting Kota and the Power of Social Media

Since then, at least 100 doctors from around the world have visited Kota to study our high-volume model of ophthalmic practice. Many of these visiting doctors come with the intention of reproducing our model at a time when funding is sparse. Still, they are confronted with many questions: How can they build a team? How can they buy or lease land? How can they reach patients? How can they build a brand image? These are the several challenges that one needs to keep in mind. In our case, we utilized the power of social media to share our articles and surgical videos and establish a global presence. We also gained worldwide respect by continuing down the path of academia, where we contributed more than 150 scientific articles in prestigious peer-reviewed ophthalmology and other medical journals.

## Fulfilling the Vision of Health for All

As our hospital became embedded in the culture of Kota and established itself, I decided it was time to fulfil another vision. I was not only working as a doctor, surgeon and academic, but also as the office bearer of several medical societies. I had served as the vice president of the Indian Medical Association (IMA), president of the Kota Division Ophthalmology Society (KDOS), editor of the *Journal of the Rajasthan Ophthalmological Society (ROS)*, and secretary of the Swasthya Seva Sanstha. These positions prepared me to fulfil my vision of a healthy society. I deeply believed that a doctor is not only a clinician or a surgeon, but also an educator responsible for creating awareness in the society for the prevention of diseases. Along with organizing several camps to create awareness about eye diseases, I doubled down on my efforts to create public awareness programmes to promote a healthy lifestyle. It was important to me that we spread the simple message that prevention is better than cure, far and wide. We organized the public awareness program (in association with Rotary Club, Lions' Club, IMA, ROS, KDOS, ROS, Swasthya Seva Sanstha, etc.) on the occasion of each and every important health day. The news about the celebration of these important health days was published prominently by the print media and also shared on social media platforms.[*] From World Health Day, World Sight Day, Doctors' Day, World Prematurity Day, World Hypertension Day, World Suicide Prevention Day to World Cancer Day, World Heart Day, World Diabetes Day, World Malaria Day, World Hepatitis Day, and World Glaucoma Week, we celebrated each and every health awareness day with the same motivation. But along with the

---

[*] For more details on these activities, please see 'Indian Medical Association (IMA) Kota Branch Activity Report by DR Suresh K Pandey, Secretary IMA Kota', Scribd. Available at: https://www.scribd.com/presentation/352184358/Indian-Medical-Association-IMA-Kota-Branch-Activity-Report-by-Dr-Suresh-K-Pandey-Secretary-IMA-Kota#.

need for prevention, I've added another layer to what constitutes healthy living, lately: scanning yourself internally.

When you meet with an accident, you undergo several tests from CT scans to X-rays, to rule out any trauma, bleeding of the internal organs, bone fractures and others. But is there a technology to scan our deepest fears and drives? Life, I have come to believe, is all about interrogating ourselves—asking questions and seeking answers. As I complete fifty-five years of my life journey, I now ask myself the tough questions: the pros and cons of my work, my responsibilities as a father, spouse, doctor, or a member of society. I asked myself: What are my top ten aspirations? What are my five biggest strengths that I would like to transfer to the next generations? What are the five achievements in my personal and professional life that I am most proud of? Who are the six personalities whom I would like to emulate as my role models? What are the dreams or goals that I wished to achieve but did not pursue for some reason? What is my action plan for my professional career for the next five or ten years? If this were to be the last year of my life, what are three wishes that I would like to fulfil within this year? What are the two things that if done consistently for six months from today, would make a significant difference in my pursuit for greater success? What are the important decisions that I am delaying? How much personal time do I invest in myself every week to understand the present and plan for the future?

I don't have all the answers but the exercise of finding answers in itself is vital to explore and evaluate the idea of yourself. It's a tough task, sometimes annoying as well. But over the past many years, I have become dutiful about following it. Writing about one's own self is among the toughest assignments because while answering these questions for myself, I often explore and rediscover new aspects of myself. It reminds me of what Anthony Robbins said, 'Successful people ask better questions, and as a result, they get better answers.'

# 24

# My Ikigai

## The Path, Vision and Formula for My Success

*'Nothing in the world can take the place of persistence. Talent will not; nothing is more common than unsuccessful men with talent. Genius will not; unsuccessful genius is almost a proverb. Education will not; the world is full of educated derelicts. Persistence and determination alone are omnipotent.'*

—Calvin Coolidge

On the first Tuesday of every month, I meet my pharma colleagues. Close to sixty medical representatives come to meet me and update me about their products. The meetings begin at 8.30 P.M. and often run on till well after midnight. I rarely sit and conduct all my meetings standing, which often makes me the butt of the jokes. I have often heard my staff and those who come to meet me, discuss in a conspiratorial style, the source of my energy. Some say it to my face: 'Your energy level is maintained regardless of the time of the day. After seeing 100–120 patients and operating on ten to twenty or sometimes thirty eyes, tiredness is still not visible on your face.' Sometimes when I respond to these observations, it appears corny, but it is the truth. My passion drives me. Does a mother get tired taking care of her children? I enjoy every moment of my work—it is what the Japanese call 'Ikigai'—one's passion and purpose in life.

In May 2015, I was in Tokyo to participate in an ophthalmology conference. I met a world-renowned eye surgeon, Dr Takayuki Akahoshi, with whom I performed live surgery during the Video Cataracta meeting in Milan, Italy, and conducted a few instructional courses during the international ophthalmology conferences. On the last day of the conference, Mahathir bin Mohamad, the former Prime Minister of Malaysia, visited Japan. While his stated primary objective was attending and appearing at conferences, he also had a more important private agenda to attend to, which was to undergo cataract surgery at Mitsui Memorial Hospital in Tokyo's Chiyoda Ward. For that operation, Mahathir relied on the world's leading authority on cataracts, Dr Takayuki Akahoshi. Dr Akahoshi was perhaps one of the fastest phaco surgeons in the world. He performs nearly sixty cataract surgeries every day. Unsurprisingly, his secret is his ikigai. He has deeply probed and contemplated his life's purpose and that has helped him chart the course of his professional life.

Understanding why we are here is a means to plan a career and a professional life effectively. Ikigai is about soul-searching. It is about asking 'What am I good at? What can I be paid for? What does the world need right now? What do I love?' It's the satisfactory responses to these questions that will effectively help you arrive at who you are and what your passion is. For me, it always comes back to the two things I am passionate about: attaining the best results for my patients and seeing them happy. This has worked for me on every single day of my twenty-five-year journey as an eye surgeon.

## A Day in My Life

I am a morning person. I wake up at about 5.30 A.M. and go cycling at 6 A.M. After one hour of working out, I get back home at 7 A.M. Cycling gives me the energy boost to start my day without feeling drowsy or fatigued. Regular exercise is an essential habit nurtured by great performers in any field. Since my days in **PGIMER**, Chandigarh, my eating patterns have been rather set. I eat a heavy breakfast, a light lunch and a lighter dinner. Throughout the day, I drink plenty of water, which maintains my energy. I also eat lots of fruits and salads. But sometimes I err, like the early days of the pandemic. In 2020, my blood pressure was constantly at 140/90 and my blood sugar was 120 mg fasting, which are both too high. I reduced my salt intake and paid attention to regular exercise. Within a few weeks, my BP and fasting sugar were back to normal. 'Let food be thy medicine and medicine be thy food,' Hippocrates had said. One can overcome most of the lifestyle diseases such as hypertension, diabetes and others with regular exercise and by paying attention to food, dietary habits, sleep patterns, etc.

My clinical day starts at about 9 A.M. This is when I see post-operative cases. Before the COVID-19 pandemic, we would see about 180 to 200 OPD cases per day and operate on fifteen to eighteen (sometimes twenty) cases, from Monday to Saturday. Many doctors who come to visit me are surprised at the high turnout at my ophthalmic practice. I am often asked how I handle these cases without feeling stressed. The answer is simple. Ophthalmology does not deal with life and death, and therefore I can afford to make my work enjoyable in most of the cases. I love interacting with my patients, making their experiences fun and engaging. I use humour and pleasantries in every interaction with them. I take interest in them, listen to them without interrupting them, and often identify and praise something unique about their personality.

One day, a retired army officer came to see me. He had an impressive handlebar moustache. I complimented him and asked him how he maintained it. The gentleman was pleased by my interest. He explained to me how he spent over an hour every day on maintaining his moustache. From his handlebar, the conversation moved to his life and family. I could see that the military man was feeling relaxed and light-hearted. He ended the consultation with a selfie with me. I was confident that he had returned home happy— and I was right. He spoke highly about our service to his friends and family and referred our services to many. He, too, would return if he needed any treatment or advice. And if on those occasions, I was busy in the OT, he would wait for as long as it took to meet me and talk to me for a few minutes. It wasn't just him. I looked forward to these interactions as they would make me forget everything that was stressing me out.

One day, a patient came to see me dressed in traditional Rajasthani gear complete with a beautiful Rajasthani turban (*pagadi*) on his head. After examining his eyes and explaining the treatment, I complimented his attire, especially the turban. The man told me how he paid special attention to tying his turban. He was a Rajput who had a close relationship with the Kota Darbar or the royal family of Kota. Incidentally, it was they who had given him this turban. 'I learned an important lesson from the royal family,' the man told me. 'People judge you within the first thirty seconds of meeting you, hence you should be Dressed in a way that they can have a good impression of you and your personality.' I adjusted my apron. The man was right.

Apart from casual, everyday conversation, I use language to connect with people. We live in a country teeming with various languages. Apart from English and Hindi, I can speak a bit of Sanskrit, Marwari, Bhojpuri, Punjabi and Bengali, so whenever patients who speak these languages meet me, I speak to them in their language. It immediately puts a smile on their face and creates a positive impression that is long-lasting. This is important in a highly stressful situation like a doctor's clinic, where laughter and a few light-hearted moments are essential to puncture the cloud of stress.

I typically operate after eating a light lunch. Most of these cases are cataracts and while some surgeries are quick, some can stake time. Each case, however, is unique and I believe in making every patient comfortable. If it is an elderly patient, I often ask them about their family and they are happy to share details. I often talk to them about their religion and discuss the Geeta or the Quran. If it's someone younger, I talk to them about their hobbies and discuss mine. By doing this, everyone feels connected and also it helps soothe their anxiety and frayed nerves. After performing surgeries, I come back to the OPD from 5–7 P.M. and after that, I return home to spend time with my daughter and my wife. By 10.30 P.M., I am in bed.

In August 2022, I celebrated my fifty-fourth birthday. It was a time of both joy and reflection. I looked back on the past sixteen years of my entrepreneurial journey—not easy, by any measure, but deeply satisfying. We have touched the lives of more than 15 lakh people and another 100,000 through our community outreach services. With four sub- and superspecialty ophthalmological services and full-fledged ancillary services, we have grown to become one of the leading eye care providers of this part of Rajasthan, India. We have successfully performed over 1 lakh eye surgeries and laser procedures. We reached out to the community by conducting over 2,000 free eye screening camps and school screening programmes. We have established a team of dedicated optometrists and have helped hundreds of families secure jobs. All along, we have continued to maintain a firm grasp over academia by training healthcare professionals and students through courses, workshops and educational videos. We have delivered over 100 lectures, published 150 papers, and provided much-needed recognition for individual contributions to the medical profession and eye care. As we complete seventeen years of restoring sight and hope to thousands of people, it is my staff and patients I must thank, as well as my collaborators, who have supported us throughout this wonderful journey. As the popular saying goes, a place is only as good as the people in it—the same is true for an organization. We are only as good as the people who work with us and support us. And in that regard, I don't hesitate in saying we are the best.

## Cycling, My Passion

Sir Arthur Conan Doyle has written, 'When the spirits are low, when the day appears dark, when work becomes monotonous, when hope hardly seems worth having, just mount a bicycle and go out for a spin down the road, without thought on anything but the ride you are taking.'

I developed a knee hematoma when I was in Moscow, while taking photographs for a group of doctors. An orthopaedic surgeon suggested surgery to drain it. Another orthopaedic surgeon told me to continue with conservative treatment and that the hematoma would absorb. I followed conservative treatment. I followed the quadriceps exercise and slowly noticed an improvement in the pain.

I took regular physiotherapy and also trained my subconscious mind. I started cycling with the motivation of Dr Ashok Moondra and Dr Bharat Singh Shekhawat. Dr Moondra came to me for his eye (pterygium and cataract) surgery and inspired me to go for cycling.

I would post an inspiring quote every week on social media as a morning motivational message involving cycling. This was liked by thousands of patients, colleagues and friends. Many young doctors, patients and pharmaceutical colleagues were inspired by these posts, especially when they noticed that I could do cycling despite having such a hectic schedule. I was considered to be a fitness freak and health enthusiast, and this led to me inspiring and motivating several friends and colleagues.

Cycling motivated me and gave me a break from my busy schedule. The creator of the *Peanuts* comic, Charles M. Schultz, wrote, 'Life is like a 10-speed bicycle. Most of us have gears we never use'.

There is plenty of scientific evidences to support that cycling (or any exercise) makes us happier. A 2010 study from the American College of Sports Medicine showed that just a thirty-minute exercise session can boost your mood and tackle depression. It comes down to the heightened production of chemicals in the brain that help to keep you happy, such as serotonin, dopamine and phenylethylamine. Not only this, but exercise releases growth hormones that increase the supply of blood and oxygen to the brain, stimulating the release of powerful mood-enhancing endorphins.

These chemical messengers can create euphoria and pain relief that is stronger than that produced by morphine. If walking for thirty minutes can act as a method for managing feelings of depression, completely free from prescribed medication in people with diagnosed depression who aren't necessarily cyclists, the principles can surely be applied to our kind, too. After all, if low-to-moderate-intensity exercise is all that is needed to give yourself a boost, imagine the benefits that cyclists can get from intense exercise such as thirty minutes of pedalling hard.

Alongside the psychological and emotional benefits of exercise, also remember that it can boost your confidence by helping you get into shape and meet exercise goals; it can take your mind off worries, increase social interaction—with like-minded cyclists—and help you feel more in control. Do you really need any more reasons to get on your bike? I think not.

# 25

# It's Between Me and God

## A Life of Miracles

*'Leap, and the net will appear.'*

—Julia Cameron

It was oppressively hot in May 1978. But the heat didn't matter. I had just finished my fifth grade examinations and was excited for the summer vacation. My family had also made plans to leave for Kanpur to attend my cousin's wedding. He was my maternal uncle's son and I had heard a lot about their family. I couldn't wait to embark on my first train journey. My mother, sister, grandfather and I boarded a train from Kota junction and reached Agra at 5 P.M. After a three-hour break, we boarded a train from Agra to Kanpur at 8 P.M. Back then, most trains were steam locomotives and had no iron grilles on the windows.

## Escaping from Kanpur's Kidnappers

At 5.30 A.M. the next day, the train halted. I was sleeping by the window and suddenly, I felt something on me. I immediately woke up and saw that someone had slipped their hands inside the window and was trying to pull me out. There was absolutely no noise around me and I was too stunned to react. My grandfather was sleeping on the berth opposite mine. Suddenly, he turned towards my window and saw that I was being pulled out. He yelled and immediately rushed towards me to pull me back. The person who wanted to kidnap me immediately ran away and disappeared within a few seconds. By God's grace, I was saved.

When my mother learnt about the incident, she was horrified. But my grandfather pacified her. At Kanpur station, when my cousin came to pick us up, my grandfather narrated the incident to him. He wasn't shocked. He told us about how criminals in the Kanpur region often kidnapped children, mutilated their bodies and sent them to beg. When I heard this, my respect for my grandfather increased tremendously. He had saved my life. I thought that this was my rebirth. If he had not saved me, I could have wound up as a child forced into begging. To this day, forty-five years later, the sensation of those arms slipping inside the train and trying to pull me out makes me break into a sweat. This was not the only time when a miracle saved my life.

## Surviving a Potentially Fatal Car Accident

It was Sunday, 8 September 2002 and I was working to finish a book on dry eye diseases. It had been commissioned by Jitendra P. Vij, CEO, Jaypee Brothers, New Delhi, to be launched at the American Academy of Ophthalmology (AAO) conference, a few weeks later. Dr Vidushi was flying to the USA for the first time after our marriage. After my stint with Professor David Apple in Charleston, I moved to John A. Moran Eye Center, Salt Lake City, Utah. I was offered the position of instructor and later on research assistant professor by Chairman Professor Randall J. Olson. I had also recently purchased a second-hand Toyota Corolla. Life seemed to be looking up.

On that fateful Sunday, I was driving to attend a lunch with some of my colleagues. But a nagging headache kept troubling me. I took a painkiller after lunch and got ready to drive back. After fifteen minutes of driving, I dozed off for a few seconds. My foot was on the accelerator and the speed was 80 miles per hour. The next thing I knew, my car had crashed into a pole on the roadside and then into a tree. The airbag flung open and I noticed an unusual smell in the cabin. My car was badly damaged but I did not have even a scratch.

As the emergency vehicle arrived at the accident site to take me to the hospital, I tried to understand what had happened. I was sleep-deprived because of the long hours I spent working. To top it off, the painkiller had added to my drowsiness. I read the warning written on the tablet strip, 'consumption of this medication can cause drowsiness', only after the accident. I heard one of the nurses from the emergency team tell me, 'Oh, lucky you! God protected you! You did not even have a scratch after such a horrible accident!' My vitals were stable. A CT scan of the head and several other tests were done to rule out internal damage or bleeding. Everything was normal. I was discharged after twenty-four hours. But my white Toyota Corolla was not as lucky. It was damaged beyond repair. The insurance company evaluated the price of my car and issued me a cheque, using which I purchased a secondhand Toyota Corolla. This one was black.

Road accidents are a major cause of mortality globally. A study from Virginia Tech Transportation revealed that 20 per cent of car crashes are caused by fatigue, with young drivers being particularly vulnerable to driving while fatigued. While I escaped an accident unscathed, my parents-in-law didn't. Once, when they were driving back home, a truck suddenly came in front of their car, causing their car to collide with the divider. It was almost past midnight. My father-in-law was crying for help desperately. A couple stopped their car, shattered my in-laws' car windows and rescued them. They had sustained only minor injuries.

'Highway hypnosis' is the state of mind that is experienced by a car driver or truck driver while driving across a long distance. This phenomenon happens only on extremely smooth and traffic-free roads. The driver feels like they are sleeping 'with eyes wide open' while driving and this is not due to the influence of any alcohol or drugs. It has been known to lead to high-speed accidents and is a major reason for the loss of several lives each year.

After surviving my own fatal accident thanks to my seatbelt and safety airbags, I always promote safe driving to all my patients, advising them to wear seatbelts and helmets, obey all traffic rules, driving within prescribed limits, avoiding talking on mobile phones while drive, avoid driving after consuming alcohol or pills that can cause drowsiness. Our entire team also participates in various road safety awareness activities during National Road Safety Week celebrated from 11 to 17 January every year.

## A Guiding Hand

It was mid-January in 1998, I had successfully completed my MS in Ophthalmology from PGIMER, Chandigarh. It was my life's biggest achievement and I was full of gratitude towards God for helping me at each and every step during this very difficult journey. I decided to visit some of the most renowned eye hospitals in India to see how they worked and explore the possibility of doing an advanced ophthalmology fellowship there. I took the train to visit the Aravind Eye Hospital, Madurai. There, I waited in the meditation room, where I saw Dr Govindappa Venkataswamy meditating. He remained still for at least half an hour. Once he got up, I greeted him and introduced myself. I told him that I had come from Chandigarh and would like to learn the secrets to become a visionary like him. He invited me into his office. As we talked in his office, he started telling me about his journey. About how the philosophy of Aravind eye care is to treat everyone, irrespective of their ability to pay. He further told me, 'Intelligence and capability are not enough. There must be the joy of doing something beautiful. When we grow with a spiritual consciousness, we identify with all that is in the world; there is no exploitation. It is ourselves we're helping, ourselves we're healing.'

I returned with overwhelming gratitude. I thought God was helping him to build the largest eye care system in the world. Dr Venkataswamy's simplicity and dedication made a tremendous impact on my mind.

After spending a week in Madurai, I visited Puttaparthi and Prasanthi Nilayam, the ashram of Sathya Sai Baba. Many renowned doctors were his devotees. Dr Eric Arnott) was one of them. A world-renowned British eye surgeon, his inner calling had brought him to India, where he donated a well-equipped eye care van to Sathya Sai Baba for helping blind people. When I took *darshan* in the evening, I felt the divine presence. I also spent three days at Sathya Sai Superspecialty Hospital. After this incredible encounter, I reached Chennai and had the opportunity to meet Dr S.S. Badrinath. Dr Badrinath had heard Kanchi Kamakoti Shankaracharya emphasize the need for a charitable eye hospital with a missionary spirit and service with dedication. Dr Badrinath and Dr Vasanti came forward and started Sankara Nethralaya from a small room. Today, Sankara Nethralaya has become a global icon in the field of eye care and retinal diseases. These experiences made me take a hard look at my career. I wondered what the purpose of life was. What was the reason some people kept on progressing in life and others did not? How does spirituality help anyone to achieve that purpose?

Even today, I don't have the answers to these questions, but rather only a collection of experiences that define me. I was a weak infant, saved by the hard work of doctors. At ten, I could have been kidnapped or killed, but my grandfather saved me. And then I thrived. I became a doctor, went to the USA, Australia, and escaped unscathed from what could have been a fatal accident. I got married, built a family, and from an initial plan to stay overseas, I returned to India and started my own practice. We didn't have the money but we had the next best thing: an indomitable spirit, and that continues to drive us to this day. When I think about all these incidents, it becomes clear to me that I was destined to live a purposeful life. Help everyone, every day; '*Atamvat Sarve Bhuteshu*' or the lesson that one should feel the happiness and distress of others as his own.

# 26

# When I Wanted to Become a Monk

*'When fear knocks on your door, send faith to answer.'*

—Joyce Meyer

In August 1990, the country was in the throes of a conflict. Prime Minister V.P. Singh had announced in Parliament that his government had accepted the Mandal Commission report, which recommended 27 per cent reservation for Other Backward Class (OBC) candidates at all levels of its services. Many upper-caste students launched nationwide protests. While agitations and demonstrations were going on in India, there was turmoil in my mind also.

## Mandal Agitation and Maha Prayan of My Spiritual Mentor

My spiritual guru, Param Poojya Gurudev, Pandit Shri Ram Sharma Acharya had left his physical body on Gayatri Jayanti (2 June 1990). In his memory, the Gayatri Pariwar, Shantikunj team, had organized a programme called 'Sankalp Shradhanjali Samaroh' in Haridwar. And this is when the turmoil within me and the outside collided. I wanted to immediately leave for Haridwar but my city, Jabalpur, was gripped with protests. Trains were being stopped by the agitating students and public property were being set on fire. It was nearly impossible to step out during that time. But I had decided to reach Haridwar and I braced myself for a difficult journey.

I remembered Gurudev and boarded a train. After fourteen hours, I reached New Delhi safely. Then I took another train for Haridwar and joined a sea of devotees who had arrived to pay their tributes to Gurudev. I listened with rapt attention as his wife, Vandiniya Mata Ji Smt. Bhagwati Devi Sharma, addressed the crowd. 'In this long, slow, tedious and meandering march of the evolution of human consciousness, culture and civilization, only rarely have avatars appeared to raise human consciousness to a higher nobler plane. Pandit Shriram Sharma Acharya, undoubtedly, belongs to this small rare group of divine *vibhutis*. Born on 20 September 1911, in the village Anwalkhera in Agra, Acharya Shri's whole life was devoted to Bhaghirath-like *tapasya* for the emergence of a new era of universal peace, harmony, and goodwill.'

I was a final-year medical student and I had had a ringside view of his very inspiring life. I saw how, from scratch and without financial power, Gurudev united millions of people to follow the path of simple living and high thinking. How when he was only fifteen years old, he endeavoured twenty-four *mahapurushcharans* of Gayatri Maha-mantra, took part in the non-violent struggle for India's independence, went to jail a number of times, and embarked upon the task of social and moral upliftment through spiritual means with the blessings of Mahatma Gandhi. A sage, visionary and social reformer, Acharya Shri propounded the 100 points of Yug Nirman Yojna for social, intellectual and spiritual evolution. He lived a simple, disciplined life full of devout austerity, visited the Himalayas several times, and attained spiritual eminence and foresight. He also translated the entire Vedic Vangmaya in lucid Hindi and accomplished the feat of writing more than 2,400 enlightening books in Hindi on all aspects of life. His writings encompass far-reaching, sagacious and feasible solutions to the innumerable problems of today.

The Gayatri Pariwar fraternity, Shantikunj Ashram (the headquarters of Gayatri Pariwar), an academy for moral and spiritual awakening; Brahmavarchas Research Institute which strives to synthesize science with spirituality, Akhand Jyoti Sansthan, Mathura, Gayatri Tapobhumi, Mathura, and thousands of social reform and sadhana centres (Gayatri Shakti Peeth) around the globe, are other grand contributions of Yugrishi Pandit Shriram Sharma Acharya to the modern world. After enlightening the lives of millions of people, Gurudev voluntarily shed his physical sheath on 2 June 1990, but even after his physical departure, the mission spread to global dimensions and forty-one Ashwamedh Yagyas (thirty-two in India, nine abroad, including the UK, the USA, Canada, Australia and South Africa) were performed to carry forward the tasks initiated by the Yugrishi.

Ever since I was a young boy, I read Gurudev's books and grew passionate about the convergence of science and spirituality. I explored spirituality further as a student in Jabalpur at Sansakar Dhani, a centre of several spiritual gurus like Osho Rajneesh, Maharishi Mahesh Yogi, and others. I visited their birthplace, their ashrams, read their biographies and was impressed by their extraordinary writing, oratory skills and spiritual abilities. At eighteen, I visited Shantikunj Haridwar and learnt more about Shri Ram Sharma Acharya, who was Sant Kabeer, Samarth Guru Ramdas, and Swami Ram Krishna Paramhansa in his past births. During these nine days of spiritual camps, I slept on the floor, woke up at 3 A.M., bathed, and sat in meditation. The meditation was in the voice of Shri Ram Sharma Acharya.

Gurudev would ask us to focus on the bodily chakras one by one and instruct us to meditate and awaken all of them. After this, we would visit the Akhand Deepak (an earthen lamp lit continuously since 1928). The first time I visited, I stayed for nine days and I would do these nine-day pilgrimages twice in a year. My last visit was in January 1990, when I got a once-in-a-lifetime opportunity to catch a glimpse of Gurudev himself. By this time, Gurudev had written a lot of revolutionary literature, even predicting future catastrophes.

'The circumstances which you are experiencing today,' Guruji said, 'will not remain tomorrow. Destruction will be everywhere. A lot of problems will come. And you will not be able to protect yourself from the problem. In all directions, when the tornado comes, when the storm comes, rain comes, no man can be safe. The coming days are going to be horrific. When diseases spread, they spread in a fashion that doctors are left saying "We haven't heard its name, we haven't seen it, we haven't been taught about it in books. What medicine should we use to treat this? What injections to inject, what medicines to provide?" These diseases will keep coming. We are surrounded by these outbursts of nature. We are surrounded by a scarcity of resources. Then, what will you do about it? We shall collect them into an axis. There will be one religion for the entire world. There will be one nation for the entire world. There will be one management, one arrangement for the entire world. The arrangement will be such that there will be no inequality. Everyone will have the right to equality. There will be no differences between people. We all shall live in unity.'*

## Why I Wanted to Become a Monk

Gurudev's departure left me aggrieved. I recalled the early days of my spirituality, specifically, a day in July 1993 when Gurudev's message written in the handwriting of Vandniya Mataji on the whiteboard, left an indelible mark on me. 'Even if there is a storm, skilled boaters bring the boat to the shore. No matter how fierce the war being fought on many fronts is, the courageous and intelligent commanders are victorious and achieve fame.' The message further

---

* Quoted from 'Coronavirus prediction| COVID-19 | Pandit Shri Ram Sharma Acharya's Prediction on Coronavirus in 1986' [video], YouTube. Available at: https://www.youtube.com/watch?v=HAGg2Q47FpA.

says: 'Those who have national interest at heart, a spirit of service and self-respect, but whose family responsibilities are not very big, should correspond with Shantikunj and think about residing here. Neither Ravana nor Sikandar's desires can be fulfilled, but no one will face any problem in the Brahminic livelihood of the average Indian citizen, consider it our assurance.'*

The message had a powerful appeal and it gained a permanent place in my mind. I was in tears and I expressed my desire to become a monk at Shantikunj Haridwar and participate in Gurudev's activities for the rest of my life. I had discussed my inner calling with Mataji and she told me to discuss it with Dr Pranav Pandya (son-in-law of Gurudev and Mataji). Dr Pandya told me to first complete MS Ophthalmology so I could help provide sight to the blind. Gayatri Mission energized and inspired me during my life's most adverse times and I decided to do as Dr Pandya advised. After completing my MS, I discussed my desire to become a monk again with Gurudev's daughter, Smt. Shail Bala Pandya. She suggested that God had given me this particular role as an eye surgeon. As a skilful eye surgeon, she explained, I could make a difference in the lives of many. She told me to continue practising as a surgeon keeping God in mind. Just as Sri Krishna tells Arjun in the *Mahabharat*, 'कर्मण्येवाधिकारस्ते मा फलेषु कदाचन । मा कर्मफलहेतुर्भुर्मा ते संगोऽस्त्वकर्मणि ॥' That is, to perform one's duty without worrying about the final outcomes or rewards.

My doubts were clear. I returned to Chandigarh and would soon leave for the USA to carry out my life's mission. I had learnt that we should perform our duties without considering the result of our righteous actions. Even if it hurts us or destroys us, we must do our duty because that's all we can do. We have no control over the result we will get from our actions. A doctor must treat, a surgeon must perform surgery, a student must learn, a soldier must fight, an

---

* *Akhand Jyoti*. April 1993. Available at: http://literature.awgp.org/akhandjyoti/1993/April/v2.52.

architect must build, a politician must make the best decisions for his people. These duties are their code. In upholding these, they may be hurt or harmed in some way; yet, they should perform their duties with good ethics, even when it may come at a personal cost. This is how society endures, and the fruit of one's action is received. But if code is broken out of a desire for personal benefits, society collapses. Your duty is your right but the fruit of your action is not.

I was ready to perform my duty ethically but I decided to continue my spiritual practice. I had a keen desire to strengthen my spiritual abilities and come close to unlocking my higher potential and that's what took me from the Rajneesh Ashram to Maharishi Mahesh Yogi Ashram to the Hare Krishna Mission. At the Hare Krishna Mission, Chandigarh, I met Narendra Agarwal, an IIT graduate who has now become known as Prabhu Narottam Das. He was only twenty-two years old and dedicated his life to the Hare Krishna Movement. I also visited Puttaparthi and was very impressed by the campus of the Sathya Sai Baba ashram. I experienced peace, tranquillity and a divine presence there. After visiting several spiritual organizations, saints and sages, several questions came to my mind: How was their personality so attractive? Why did so many followers have such a strong faith in them? How were they so influential? Could I become like them?

As I pondered over these questions, I realized that their enlightenment stemmed from within them; from their 'third eye' chakra (located just below your belly button), Solar plexus chakra, Heart chakra, Throat chakra, Third eye chakra, Crown chakra. During my stay at Shantikunj, I used to meditate every morning with Gurudev's voice to awaken the seven chakras of the body. These include Root chakra (located at the base of your spine), Sacral or Svadhisthana. The Third Eye Chakra, also called the *Ajna* Chakra, is the centre of perception, consciousness and intuition. Pronounced 'Agya Chakra', it is the focal point of concentration during asana or meditation practices. The Third Eye Chakra is located between the eyebrows, at the centre of your head, and unlike the two physical eyes which see the past and the present, the third eye reveals insight into the future. This chakra establishes a connection with the external world through inner vision. Focusing on the third eye is believed to motivate us to move beyond worldly desire and distractions. When the Ajna Chakra is awakened, it increases consciousness and transcends to a higher realm. During my experience of nine days of spiritual camps at Shantikunj and visits to several places, I came to the conclusion that it's the activation of this 'third eye' that is spirituality's toughest conquest. To achieve this, you have to conquer *Kama* or bodily desires, *Krodha* or anger, as well as greed, jealousy, pride, as well as attachment. It's when we do this—when we find love within ourselves, when we become content, generous and fearless, that we come close to awakening the third eye. It's a pursuit for life—of life.

# 27

# Giving Back to Society and
# Leaving a Legacy

Philanthropists and social contributions have always been central to my practice. I am constantly inspired by the legacies left behind by some of the personalities I have been fortunate enough to cross paths with, and here, also mention some people whose lives I have been able to play a part in changing, either through our hospital or in a personal capacity. On 30 March 1996, Dr Gullapalli Nageswara Rao visited PGIMER, Chandigarh as a guest speaker at a conference of the International Association of Contact Lens Educators. Late Dr Jagjit Singh Saini introduced Dr Rao, who was an internationally renowned and well-respected ophthalmologist, working as an associate professor at the University of Rochester, Rochester, NY, United States. He returned to India to found the L.V. Prasad Eye Institute (LVPEI) in Hyderabad. Every one of us was very curious to know the details of what motivated him to give up his academic career and return to India to start from scratch.

The next day, while meeting Dr Rao, I asked him this question. He smiled and answered that it is the ability to make a difference (MAD). India has the highest number of blind/visually impaired people in the world and his services are needed here. He also shared the story of how the institute was founded. In the beginning, before the brick and mortar institute came into being, the renowned Indian filmmaker Sri Akkineni Lakshmi Vara Prasad Rao, popularly known as L.V. Prasad, decided to invest a part of the profits of his blockbuster film *Ek Duje Ke Liye* for a worthy cause. He donated ₹1 crore and five acres of land for establishing the state-of-the-art eye institute. In recognition of this gesture, the board of the institute decided to name the institute after him. Over the years, his family has continued to support the institute's work. His son, Mr Ramesh Prasad, Managing Director of Prasad Film Laboratories, is a founder trustee of LVPEI and is the longest-serving member of the Hyderabad Eye Institute's governing board, along with Dr Rao. Since its inception in 1987, the mission of LVPEI has been to provide 'equitable and efficient eye care to all sections of society'. LVPEI has served nearly 23.8 million people, with over 50 per cent of them entirely free of cost, irrespective of the complexity of care needed. The institute trained more than 5,000 eye doctors and 10,000 ophthalmic assistants from India and overseas. This is an example of how a contribution to society can make a huge difference.

I was very much inspired by the example of L.V. Prasad Eye Institute and the story of Dr G.N. Rao. He went out of his comfort zone, leaving the cushy lifestyle of a prestigious university in the USA. He wanted to make a difference by returning to India and want to give back to society, which earned him great respect, through teaching, training ophthalmic surgeons and providing free eye treatment to people below the poverty line.

Since my childhood, I was very much influenced by people making a positive contribution to society. I also wanted to become a doctor who worked on many fronts. A healer, who could heal patients through treatment, a social reformer, a fitness freak, environmentally conscious, a motivator, a philanthropist and a family man. My job as an eye surgeon helped me to achieve this, to a great extent.

It was the beginning of the new year, on 2 January 2016, and Dr Vidushi and I were returning from Jaipur to Kota by road. On the way, we slowed down our vehicle as it started raining. About 40 kms before reaching Kota, we noticed one homeless lady by the road. She appeared very weak, with long hair and her clothes were raggedy. We stopped our vehicle and in order to help her, we called our staff to reach the spot with water and food and some warm clothes. Our staff reached her after forty-five minutes and gave her warm clothes and food. Perhaps, she was a patient of psychiatric illness and living on the road, surviving on whatever food was given to her by the passers by. This was winter time and there was a cold wave. We made a few phone calls to Mother Teresa Home, Apna Ghar Ashram and other shelter homes.

Within a few hours, the Apna Ghar Ashram team reached the spot and she was admitted to Apna Ghar Ashram, Kota. The next day, she underwent a medical examination and was found to be pregnant. When we visited Apna Ghar Ashram during the weekend, we were impressed that the same lady appeared to be doing a lot better after washing her hair, wearing new clothes, taking a bath and dressing her wounds. Talking to Dr C.S. Sushil (who was regularly giving her his time), she was suffering from mental illness (schizophrenia) and had shown improvement after being treated with antipsychotic drugs. After a few weeks, she gave birth to a male child. Both mother and child have been living happily in Apna Ghar Ashram for the past few years.

This incident left a great impact on our minds. Dr Vidushi and I were very impressed with the prompt services delivered by Apna Ghar Ashram. We both decided to become life members of their organization. We started celebrating our birthdays, wedding anniversaries, and the birth and death anniversaries of our family members with the residents of Apna Ghar Ashram. I was very curious to know their story and we decided to meet the founders and help in some way to run these services.

## Story of Apna Ghar Ashram

In 2000, Dr Brij Mohan Bharadwaj and Dr Madhuri Bharadwaj established the Apna Ghar Ashram in Bajhera village, Bharatpur district, Rajasthan. Today, this home for the homeless serves more than 5,000 people. While discussing with Dr Bhardwaj how he was motivated to start Apna Ghar Ashram, he narrated to us a story.

In his childhood, he was moved by the death of an eighty-five-year-old man named Chiranjee Baba in his native Sahroi village of Aligarh Uttar Pradesh. Chiranjee Baba had never married and lived alone in the village. He grazed everyone's cattle, and in return was fed and clothed. When he fell and injured himself, no one came to help him. Eventually, in a month, his wounds festered and he died. It's not that nobody wanted to help him. Everyone did. But they held back from taking responsibility, afraid it would fall on their plates. People will help, if someone takes responsibility and shows others how they can help.

Too young at the time to do anything about it, Dr Bhardwaj remembers wanting to help but being wary of Chiranjee Baba's sickness. His unease slowly changed into a determination to help the sick and to be able to act and save lives. Dr Madhuri was in Class 9 when she became friends with Dr Bharadwaj. They travelled from their villages every day to Aligarh. She went to her school, while he went to college. On the bus, they discussed a topic unusual for two teenagers from two small villages in Uttar Pradesh—they talked about their shared dream of leading a meaningful life, dedicated to helping those in need. They planned to become partners in this venture. Dr Brij Mohan and Dr Madhuri got married on 8 December 1993, and got ready to work on their dream. However, they decided to never have their own children as they wanted to invest all their energy in taking care of the sick and homeless. They both became doctors and brought abandoned sick people from the streets into their homes. They went a step further and announced to their shocked families that they would not have children so that they could take care of hundreds of other children.

Today, Apna Ghar Ashram takes in anyone who needs medical help, be it a child, an adult, or even an animal. Those that are sick and seem to be without any succour on the streets, are referred to Apna Ghar Ashram. Everybody who comes to Apna Ghar Ashram is treated as Prabhu ji (God), because 'they are here to teach us how to be good people'. In the span of the last five years, they have admitted 103 women who were pregnant at the time of their admission into Apna Ghar Ashram. Several of them were mentally challenged, couldn't speak or hear, and usually begged on the streets. Some of them were raped and had been abandoned by their families.

Currently, there are 86 children at Apna Ghar who were born to these abandoned or helpless women rescued from the streets. Every day, helpless people are rescued from the streets, brought to the house and given medical attention. If someone requires more specialized help, that patient is taken to the right doctor and treated. Over time, they are rehabilitated, and if possible, reunited with their families.

Dr Madhuri and Dr B.M. Bhardwaj have chosen a noble path to help the truly vulnerable, and they remain an inspiration for me and thousands of others on how to live a meaningful life. My father-in-law also shared the story of Apna Ghar when I had the opportunity to travel to Kasison to attend the school annual function and scholarship distribution program together with him. I recalled the struggles of his childhood and how he travelled to his village Kasison a few times every year, to encourage children to study. My mother-in-law Smt. Sudha Sharma donated ₹5 lakhs to construct a room at Apna Ghar Ashram in memory of my father-in-law Late Gp. Capt. (Retired) K. M. Sharma.

## Empowering the Girl Child: The Story of Laxmi Sharma

It was December 2011, Laxmi Sharma, a nineteen-year-old girl, had been introduced to us by one of our patients. She had migrated from a village near Aligarh, Uttar Pradesh. Her father was a cook and worked in a mess. Her entire family of eight members was staying in a small room. Laxmi was teaching school kids and trying hard to support the family while her father was unable to work as a cook and support his family due to a frozen shoulder and several other health issues. She passed her Class 11 with first division and wanted to pursue graduation in science and become a teacher, as teaching was her passion.

Due to the financial crisis as a result of her parent's health issues, she was unable to pay her fees, so she could not continue her studies. She spent an entire year cooking food for family members and teaching poor children in her spare time without charging any fees. Her parents were not keen on educating her as she was a girl and was 'paraya dhan', and would go to her in-laws' after her marriage anyway. When we came to know about this, we immediately paid her fees and provided money to buy books to restart her studies.

Laxmi also started teaching our daughter Ishita. She does each and every small task in a perfect way. My father- and mother-in-law treat Laxmi like their own grandchild. They always believe in empowering the girl child, as they did with Dr Vidushi. Laxmi passed BSc with honours and also received a gold medal. Later, she completed her MSc (Botany) with flying colours. She started teaching at a renowned coaching institute of Kota (Vibrant Academy). In December 2020, she got married and is now happily sharing family responsibility, while also teaching and motivating underprivileged children.

## Inaugurating a School in My Village: Late Shri Kameshwar Prasad Pandey Library

On 14 March 2022, I was invited to inaugurate Adarsh Vidhya Mandir School at Eklingpura, near Mohna. I accepted the invitation and participated in the programme wholeheartedly. It was an emotional moment for me, making the journey to visit a village (adjoining my own village, Mohna) as a chief guest, where I had once studied and played. I was impressed by the cultural programme presented by the school children. I decided to make my own small contribution by donating ₹2.5 lakhs to the school to start a library. The school authority decided to name the library after my father, Late Shri Kameshwar Prasad Pandey, as my father considered his books to be his most valuable possessions. In my speech as the chief guest, I recalled my own journey that I took as a student thirty-five years back.

## Late Pandit Brij Bhushan Lal Tiwari Scholarship

My maternal grandfather, Pandit Brij Bhushan Lal Tiwari, worked in the Indian Army and after a short service commission, he became a school teacher at Chhipabarod, district Baran, Rajasthan. At that time, doctors were not available and he also took training as an Ayurvedic practitioner for several months to help villagers free of cost. He would teach poor meritorious students and help them to pay their fee asking for nothing in return. We have heard several stories of his dedication to work, kindness and compassion by some senior citizens and his students. We recently started the Pandit Brij Bhushan Lal Tiwari Scholarship in his honour for the brightest student of Chhipabarod School securing the highest marks in the board examinations.

## Musaddi Lal Bhardwaj Scholarship at Kasison, Aligarh

My father-in-law Group Capt. [(Retd.)] K.M. Sharma started a scholarship in his own village Kasison (District Kher, Aligarh) in memory of his father, Late Shri Musaddi Lal Bhardwaj. He would go every year (for twenty years) to distribute the scholarship to school children who were financially impoverished but had an excellent academic record. Smt. Sudha Sharma, Dr Vidushi Sharma, Shri Manohar Lal Sharma accompanied him few times. He also motivated these children to excel in their studies. When he was in school, he wanted to study. He studied at Aligarh Muslim University (AMU) and faced grave financial crisis. He saved every penny to support himself, even teaching a few students every evening in exchange for a few hundred rupees.

## Giving Gift of Sight to a Mother and Child

During the past sixteen years, the team of SuVi Eye Hospital, Kota has performed more than 2,000 eye surgeries free of cost for needy people. I would like to share the story of a twenty-eight-year-old woman (Banasi Devi) and her four-year-old daughter (Teena Kumari), both of whom were rendered needlessly blind from cataract. The woman was married off at an early age, and her only child suffered from congenital cataracts. While cataract surgery is done in many free eye camps all over India, congenital cataracts are often neglected due to lack of awareness, illiteracy and poor socioeconomic condition, lack of support from family members, fear and anxiety. She and her only child were unable to seek treatment for the same and continued their life with very poor vision, and gradually they were confined to their hut, unable to perform daily activities due to lack of sight.

I happened to visit the campus of Chambal Fertilizer and Chemical Limited (CFCL) in Gadepan (situated on NH27 about 40 kms from Kota) during an eye checkup camp in December 2012. While returning to Kota, I was requested by a village head (Sarpanch) if I could examine a mother and child who had no vision, at their hut. I accepted his request and visited their hut, and was shocked to see them almost totally blind due to cataracts in this day and age! The family was extremely poor and illiterate, and it was a challenge to convince them to come for cataract surgery. Seeing their condition, I decided not to waste any more time, took help of the village head and other villagers to convince them to come for a detailed examination and brought them to the hospital in my car. After comprehensive counselling and thorough ocular and systemic investigations, I operated on both of them without any charges. The surgery was quite difficult due to the small pupil, zonular dehiscence and pre-existing posterior capsule defect, but both of them had significant improvement in vision and could actually see each other for the first time!

The child is now fifteen years old and studying in Class 9 and the mother is ably taking care of her child. Teena wants to become a school teacher in future and would like to teach poor girls free of cost. It was a life-changing experience for both mother and child, and the mother asked me if they could, in celebration of the Rakshabandhan festival, tie a Rakhi (sacred thread) on his wrist. This emotional request was accepted by him and they have been visiting us every year for the last five years to tie me a Rakhi and express their gratitude. It was also a life-changing experience for me to visit the patient and her daughter confined to their hut (due to vision problem) and witness the positive change that was seen in their life after their eye surgery.

## Morning Motivational Message with Cycling

I started cycling five years back. I made a social media page 'Morning Motivational Messages with Cycling', which has connected more than 1 lakh people to be motivated to save the environment and pursue a healthy lifestyle through cycling. I have shared more than 100 motivational videos there. These videos talk about health, happiness and healthy habits. Thousands of my patients, their family members and pharma colleagues felt motivated to start living a healthy life after watching these videos.

## Tobacco and Alcohol De-addiction

Every year, on May 31, we celebrate 'No Tobacco Day'. Our staff, together with our patients, take the pledge to avoid tobacco and other addictions. Together with several NGOs and medical organizations, we have also organized Nasha Mukti programmes to create awareness about tobacco addiction in society. We have seen more than 15 lakh patients during seventeen years of my ophthalmology practice. I had performed surgery on more than 1 lakh patients. While interacting with our patients who are addicted to tobacco and alcohol, I have asked them to leave their bad habits as they are injurious to health. My team and I have helped more than 3,000 patients overcome tobacco and alcohol addiction.

## Leaving a Legacy

As Shannon L. Alder writes, 'Carve your name on hearts, not tombstones. A legacy is etched into the minds of others and the stories they share about you.' Most of us are familiar with Stephen Covey's obituary exercise. He asks the reader to imagine their own funeral. Then, they are to ask themselves questions like: Who would give a eulogy at my funeral? What will they miss about me? What positive attributes will they associate with me? How are they describing me?

As mentioned by Steve Saint, 'Your story is the greatest legacy that you will leave to your friends. It's the longest-lasting legacy you will leave to your heirs.' I would be pleased to be a healer in yet another life. Working as an eye doctor gave me the opportunity to treat not only eye-related patients but also to interact, learn from my patients, do social work, make a difference in the life of blind or visually impaired people, inspire and leave behind a legacy for everyone, including medical students and young doctors to follow the path of care, kindness and compassion.

28

# Visualizing the Last Journey

*'Analysis of death is not for the sake of becoming fearful but to appreciate this precious lifetime.'*

—Dalai Lama

On 19 August 2019, at about 10 A.M., my father, Shri Kameshwar Prasad Pandey, was on his way to Rawatbhata to complete his pension formalities. He was keen to visit his former workplace and meet his friends. While he was waiting outside the garage for our driver to take out the car, he suddenly lost consciousness. The driver came rushing to get me and I immediately ran towards Babuji. We rushed him to a hospital and I noticed that his fist was clinched and he was having difficulty releasing the bag he was holding in his hands. He was admitted in the Intensive Care Unit and as time progressed, his condition deteriorated.

A computerized tomography (CT) scan of his head revealed massive intracranial bleeding. His condition continued to deteriorate and very soon, he was put on a ventilator. An emergency surgery called craniotomy, which requires opening the skull to drain the blood collected inside, was done by a reputed neurosurgeon to ease the pressure on the brain. But none of these measures helped.

After thirty-six hours, he passed away on 20 August 2019. I am very grateful to Dr Deepak Wadhwa (a neurosurgeon) for all his efforts in trying to save my father's life.

We could not believe he would depart so quickly as he was perfectly healthy, without any history of diabetes or hypertension, even at the age of eighty years. We brought him home at 11 P.M. on 20 August 2019 and lay his body in his room. As we sat near him, awake the entire night, I visualized his life, his contribution, his work, and his final journey. I also visualized my own last journey. Author Robin Sharma's words came to my mind: 'Who will cry when you die?'

My father told me many times, 'Son, when you were born, you cried while the world rejoiced. Live your life in such a way that when you die, the world cries while you rejoice.' As I recalled my father's life like a film, I took note of how he was determined to provide the best education to his four children despite the severe financial challenges. He was born on August 24, 1938, in Pura, Ballia, and spent his time collecting and reading motivational books, and dictionaries and increasing his knowledge and vocabulary. He would always say that motivational and self-help books are like a 'living God' and reading them would give you instant knowledge and wisdom. He always motivated us to stay happy, work like a 'Karmayogi' and always help others in life. My father was a voracious reader and firmly believed in simple living and high thinking. He motivated hundreds of his poor students to excel at their studies and also supported them financially so they could pay their fees, buy books and meet other expenses. When such students would come to meet him, they would touch his feet and express their gratitude for his teachings and financial support. My father possessed an extraordinary memory and remembered the entire *Ramayana* and quotes from various other books he read. He would surprise his colleagues and thousands of students by repeating their date of birth, weddings, and names of their family members correctly.

During the condolence meeting in his honour, many of his colleagues and students shared stories from the time they had spent with him, how he told his friends that he was proud of his children. I said a silent prayer of gratitude that in his final days, I was back home in India. My father wanted to become a doctor and because his own dream to become one remained unrealized, it gave him immense pleasure when I fulfilled his dream. It was very satisfying for him to see all the progress that I had made—not just with respect to our hospital, but also as an eye surgeon. My father experienced firsthand how surgery could lead to excellent recovery, when I performed his cataract operation and implanted AcrySof IQ ReSTOR multifocal lens in both his eyes.

My journey was especially remarkable to him because although I was born a weak child and had suffered from neonatal jaundice, I worked hard and did all I could to make my life a success. My grandfather was my inspiration, and my father did everything he could to channelize that inspiration in the right direction. In most cases, he led by example. My father often expressed his wish to donate his body to a medical college. But he passed away before he could sign the required form. Babuji also told me of his desire to donate his corneas. After his cataract surgery and an implantation of multifocal lenses, his eyesight was excellent. He was able to see clearly from a distance and read without glasses. He had filled out an eye donation pledge and as per his wish, we donated his eyes to the Eye Bank Society of Rajasthan (EBSR), Kota Chapter.

As I sat next to him on that fateful night, I recalled the great sense of accomplishment he felt in his final days. His four children are well-settled and doing much better than he or anyone in our family could have expected. But I also wondered, will my dreams be fulfilled? Would I be as satisfied during my final days? Would I be able to overcome my limitations or my shortcomings? I still had a long way to go. As an entrepreneur and director of SuVi Eye Hospital, Dr Vidushi and I have had the opportunity to embark on a deeply fulfilling journey—one that started with refusing a job. It taught me that life is too short to hold a grudge—professionally or personally.

My father didn't inherit his due from my grandfather. It could have been a lifelong pain point, but he believed that his children would do so well that property inherited by others would pale in comparison to our success. 'I raised my four children in difficult and adverse conditions,' he would say. 'Like the Pandavas, they've excelled.'

Sometimes, opportunities are purely accidental. Dr Vidushi and I were about to join the prestigious eye institute in Hyderabad but were compelled to change our plans at the last moment. This made our journey tougher but infinitely sweeter. As I recall the incident today after seventeen years, I am thankful to Professor Ravi Thomas for his help.

And sometimes, trauma and pain might be too much to ignore but the delete button should be kept handy. My father would say that the most important button on the keyboard is the delete button. He always insisted on deleting unpleasant memories and bad experiences. In life, all of us have many unpleasant stories and experiences that can sour our experience, we should learn to delete them and stop them from preventing our progress.

Most of us take life for granted; we forget that death is inevitable. We happily waste our time on meaningless things just to regretfully beg for life on the deathbed. It is always the near-death experiences that motivates us to treasure life. So instead of waiting until death, why don't we face it now? I think we should think about death and use that as a prism to rethink our priorities. If you've built your life based on other people's opinions, you will regret it. Change your perspective, and you will realize that the life that you once thought you weren't good enough to have, the life that we once labelled as 'unrealistic', was actually a life we were meant to have.

My father would say, once you wake up in the morning, you should thank God as every day is a new birth, a new beginning. 'If you live each day as if it were your last, someday you will most certainly be right.' This left an impression on me and since then, for the past decade, I have looked in the mirror every morning and asked myself, 'If today were the last day of my life, would I want to do what I'm about to do today?' And, whenever the answer has been 'no' for too many days in a row, I know I need to change something.

## My Mother

While I was in the process of sending this book for publication, my mother, Smt. Maya Devi Pandey suffered a brain stroke (thalamic bleeding) on 29 January 2023. She lost consciousness and was admitted to the ICU at Kota Heart Institute. She was a devotee of Lord Hanuman and left us for the infinite journey on 6 April 2023, on the occasion of Hanuman Jayanti. My mother has been my rock and I consider myself very fortunate to be able to seek her blessings almost every day for the past ten years. My biggest achievement has not only been serving thousands of patients in this part of India but also taking care of both my parents until the end.

My mother was born on 7 May 1945, at Chhipabarod. Her father (Late Brij Bhushan Lal Tiwari) was a schoolteacher and an Ayurvedic healer. After her education, she also wanted to become a schoolteacher to inspire girls to realize their complete potential. She was approached by the village Pradhan (Late Shri Kishan Lal Gupta) several times with an offer to work as a teacher in a village government school in Mohna. However, my paternal grandmother, who was very conservative and believed that her daughter-in-law should not step out of the house to work, shot down the prospect each time. My mother regretted not fighting against the decision but she didn't let it affect our upbringing. She protected all her children from harm not only during our childhood, but even went so far as to convince my father to leave the village to enable us to pursue higher studies and keep us shielded from all the negativity at home. She taught us the value of a never-say-die attitude and encouraged us to work hard to put smiles on the faces of our patients. Many times, she played the role of both father and mother, due to my father's introverted nature.

Remembering that I would be dead soon is the most important tool I have ever encountered to help me make the big choices in life. Death is the only certainty in life. Each one of us has witnessed losing our close family members and friends. But that's not the only death we have to face in life. Almost everything—external expectations, pride, fear of embarrassment or failure—these things just fall away in the face of death, leaving behind only what is truly important. As I visualize my own death, I am acutely aware of leaving behind a legacy. That is also the purpose of this book. To share my journey—failures, achievements and limitations—with the world. To help millions of medical students, doctors and people at large do well in life despite their fears. To do as Swami Vivekananda advised: 'Arise, awake, and not stop till you achieve the goal.'

# Afterword

Dear Reader,

First of all, please accept my sincere thanks for reading my memoir. I have shared the story of my life across three continents—India, the USA, Australia; my struggles, my successes, and my failures, as honestly as I could. I hope you enjoyed reading about my life's journey from an impoverished Indian village to the magnificent world stage of ophthalmology.

But what was the purpose of writing this memoir? What is my message?

First of all, I want to encourage you to know your passion and decide whether you really want to come out of your comfort zone to taste success or not. There are no free lunches in life and there is a price for everything—including success—which you must be prepared to pay. Sacrifices, sleepless nights, stepping out of your comfort zone, envy, spite, stress, smart and hard work, raising the bar frequently, failures, frustrations—the list is endless for those who want success. The majority of the people in this world are happy within their comfort zone and decide early in life that it is not worth it—that it is simply not their cup of tea. They decide that a laidback lifestyle is what suits them best, and they are fine with it. In other words, they are happy with whatever they are able to achieve while staying within their comfort zone.

However, there are few—less than 1 per cent—who like to take risks, push the boundaries, set higher and higher targets for themselves, and desire to establish a legacy that's not as impermanent as their time on this earth. I wrote my memoir keeping the latter in mind and thinking about how I could enrich such people's journeys with my story. The fact that you cared to pick up and read this book shows that you belong to this group of people.

Ultimately, I believe that success is due to many factors, deeds and even destiny. On the top of the list are the family environment and social circumstances in which you are placed in life. It was fate that led a village boy who walked barefoot, studied under lanterns, survived on one meal a day, and faced several other harsh realities of life early on, but was determined with a never-say-die attitude, to become a saviour of vision for so many. Surrounded by so many adversities, success is also about seeing the light at the end of a dark tunnel and seizing and making full use of the opportunities that come our way.

While pursuing my journey as an eye surgeon, I also learned early in life that one can wear multiple hats: a healer, counsellor, researcher, teacher, administrator, philanthropist, fitness freak, spiritual seeker, social reformer and motivational speaker. The important thing is to focus on the job at hand. In this book, I have tried to share what I think are the basic qualities needed for anyone to succeed: persistence, passion, focus, resilience, hard work, faith, the courage to dream big, peer pressure and support, sharing and collaboration with others and, above all, ethics, integrity and finding your own Ikigai. All these are essential ingredients if one were to write a recipe for success.

Last but not the least, remember that life comes full circle. With this book, the dreams of a village boy who read the success stories of doctors and wanted to become like one of them are being fulfilled. I hope you enjoyed reading this memoir as much as I enjoyed constantly paving the path for a journey worth writing about, and then writing it. Finally, I also hope that my journey will inspire you to write the story of your own success, years from now.

I welcome your valuable suggestions, your experiences and constructive criticism to improve the next edition of my book.

# Acknowledgements

The herculean task of writing and compiling a book of such a magnitude is not possible without the help of several people. I am very fortunate to be surrounded by so many people who make me feel blessed, cherished and fulfilled; who share my dreams and make me feel alive. It is not possible to mention each and every one of their names here. I take this opportunity to thank all of them who not only supported me in the writing of my memoir, but played an important role in facilitating my journey from a small village to becoming a doctorpreneur. To start with, I would like to acknowledge the valuable assistance and contribution of my wife, Dr Vidushi Sharma. I offer deep gratitude also to my adorable daughter, Ishita, who thoroughly understands her Papa's passion for writing and held on bravely even when I was away for the past few weeks for this project.

My sincere thanks to Professor (Dr.) Amod Gupta for writing the foreword in this book. I would like to express my deepest gratitude to Ms Apekshita Varshney, my editor, for her most valuable assistance in each and every step of this book. My most sincere thanks and gratitude to Dipankar Mukherjee and Indrani Ganguly for their editorial help and invaluable suggestions.

I would like to thank my parents and family members for their constant support and encouragement. These include Late Kameshwar Prasad Pandey, Smt. Maya Devi Pandey, Smt. Usha Pandey, Dr Rajesh Kumar Pandey, Dr Dinesh Kumar Pandey, Group Capt. (retired) Late Sh K.M. Sharma, Smt. Sudha Sharma, Shri Manohar Lal Sharma, Smt. Sadhna Sharma, etc.

My sincere thanks to all my respected teachers at Mohna, Eklingpura, Rawatbhata, Rampura, for their invaluable teachings. Namely, Shri Balvir Singh, Shri Laxmi Narayan Gupta, Shri Ramgopal Gupta, Shri Laxmi Chand Sharma, Shri Mangilal Suthar, Shri Mangilal Dashora, Shri Banshi Lal Purohit, Shri Samrathmal Jain, Late Shri Nemi Chand Nalvaya, Shri Padam Kumar Gangwal, Shri Radheshyam Namdev, Shri Rajkumar Sharma, Shri Latif Husain, Shri Arvind Kumar Lakkad, Dr M.S. Namjoshi, etc. Special thanks to all my respected teachers and alumni of NSCB Medical College, Jabalpur, M.P. These include Anatomy- Dr T.M. Garg, Dr Malviya, Dr S.K. Verma Sr, Dr S.K. Verma Jr, Dr S.K. Shrivastva, Dr Asha Dixit, Dr V. Lakhanpal, Dr P.C. Jain, Physiology- Dr B.B.L. Mathur, Dr S.S. Mishra Sr, Dr S.S. Mishra Jr, Dr R.S. Pandey, Biochemistry- Late Dr Kiran. Hasija, Dr R.K. Bidwai, Dr R. Bodke, Pathology- Dr M.A. Hafeez, Dr G.S. Chauhan, Dr J.C. Gupta, Dr Saroj Munjal, Dr Murli Krishnan, Dr Laxman Patel, Dr Sharad Jain, Dr Rajni Vishnoi, Dr A. Sant, Dr Savita Verma, Dr R.K. Jain, Dr Sanjay Totade, Dr V. Gandagule, Forensic Medicine- Dr D.K. Sakalley, Dr Trilok Mohan, Pharmacology- Dr R.K. Gupta, E.N.T.- Dr K. R. Munjal, Dr M. Tankwal, Dr Rakesh Shukla, Dr Anil Agrawal, Ophthalmology- Dr Ashok K. Mukherjee, Dr (Mrs) M. Shrivastava, Dr Vijay Bhaisare, P.S.M. Dr (Mrs) Indra Dutt, Dr David Park, Dr Pradeep Kasar, Surgery- Dr J.P. Kapoor, Dr J.K. Tandon, Dr V.K. Bhatnagar, Dr M.P. Gupta, Dr Dhananjay Sharma, Dr K.D. Baghel, Dr V.K. Raina, Dr Anil Mishra, Dr L.P. Verma, Dr Ashutosh Soni, Medicine- Dr Surinder Singh, Dr B.N. Srivastava, Dr Vivek Johari, Dr V.K. Mehta, Dr G.P. Vyas, Dr

Shashank Gupta, Dr V.D. Singh, Dr J.K. Parashar, Dr G.S. Mehta, Dr R. Trivedi, Dr B.M. Tejwani, Dr R.S. Sharma, Dr M.S. Johri, Dr Vaidhya, Gynaecology- Dr Bhatnagar, Dr R. Shrivastav, Dr V. Deshpande, Dr H. Subedar, Dr R. Chouhan, Dr A. Lele, Dr S. Khare, Paediatrics- Dr K.K. Kaul, Dr Maya Chansoria, Dr Benu Mukherjee, Dr D.K. Shrivastav, Dr Neena Patel, Orthopaedics- Dr H.K.T. Raza, Anesthesia- Dr K.P. Chansoriya, Dr B.P. Singh, Dr Ira Chandra, Dr S.K. Kriplani, Dr Atul Dixit, Radiology- Dr B.M. Arora, Dr Amarjeet Kaur, Dr S. Vale, Dr Arun Sharma, Dr A.S. Rathore, Dr Vijya Mehta, Dr Kirar, Dr Kriplani, etc.

My most sincere thanks to all faculty members and alumni of Advanced Eye Centre, PGIMER, Chandigarh. These include Dr Amod Gupta, Dr Jagat Ram, Late Dr Jagjit Singh Saini, Dr Mangat R. Dogra, Dr Arun Kumar Jain, Dr Kanwar Mohan, Dr S.S. Pandav, Dr Ashok Sharma, Dr Usha Singh. Special thanks to my seniors, friends and colleagues, Dr Vishali Gupta, Dr Neeraj Sood, Dr Mrinal Anand, Dr Ritu Lal, Dr Sangeet Mittal, Dr Suresh Kumar, Dr Subina Narang, Dr Vandana Siroha, Dr Paramjit Singh Jora, Dr Prashant Sahare, Dr Raj Anand, Dr K.B. Viswanadh, Dr Amit Gupta, Dr Shristi Raj, Dr Somesh Gupta, Dr Rakesh Jindal, Dr Dheeraj Kamra, Dr Nishith Bhardwaj, Dr Kamlesh Chandel, Dr Man Singh Chandel, etc.

I thankfully appreciate help and assistance of my mentors and colleagues during my time in the USA and Australia. These include Late Dr David J. Apple, Dr Randall J. Olson, Dr M. Edward Wilson, Dr M. Millicent W. Peterseim, Dr Geoffrey F. Tabin, Dr Nick Mamalis, Dr Liliana Werner, Dr Leonardo P. Werner, Dr Kensaku Miyake, Dr Okihiro Nishi, Dr Reijo J. Linnola, Dr Andrea M. Izak, Dr Ehud I. Assia, Dr Gerd U. Auffarth, Dr Manfred R. Tetz, Dr Qun Peng, Dr Mike P. Holzer, Dr Luis G. Vargas, Dr Josef M. Schmidbauer, Dr Robert J. Schoderbek Jr., Dr Guy Kleinmann, Late Dr Alan S. Crandall, Dr Rupal H. Trivedi, Dr Bradley S. Daines, Dr Tamer A. Mackey, Dr Stella N. Arthur, Dr Helga P.

Sandoval, Dr Tanja Rabsilber, Dr Surendra Basti, Dr Marcella Escobar-Gomez, Dr Kerry D. Solomon, Dr David T. Vroman, Dr Nithi Visessook, Dr Irmingard M. Neuhann, Dr Enrique Roig-Melo, Dr E. John Milverton, Dr Anthony J. Maloof, Dr Gagan Khannah, Dr Iain Dunlop, Dr John W. McAvoy and Dr Paul Mitchell.

My sincere thanks to the doctors and staff members of SuVi Eye Institute & Lasik Laser Center, Kota—Dr S.K. Gupta, Dr Nipun Bagrecha, Dr Deepesh Chhablani, and for their assistance. I would like to thank Dr Saurabh Savaria, Dr Randhir Jha, Dr Meenal Gupta, Dr Garima Lakhotia, Dr Arun Pandey, Dr Bharti Ahuja, Dr Nimisha Vijay, Dr Monika Nagar and all team members who worked with us and supported us during our early years. Special thanks to Dr Sujatha Sharma, Dr V. Mohan, Dr A. Sampath, Dr Kamal Mawahar, Dr Abhishek R. Kothari, Dr Manoj Sreenivasan, Dr Santosh Kumar for their inputs on the content of the book.

I would like to thank the thousands of patients, their families, the optometrists, the doctors and the hospital staff for their invaluable support in my professional life. Last but not the least, I am indebted to my publisher Penguin Random House India (Ankit Juneja and Sameer Mahale) and editor Udyotna Kumar; all medical aspirants, medical students, my patients and my friends and well-wishers who share my dreams and motivate me to do better in the future.

# About the Author

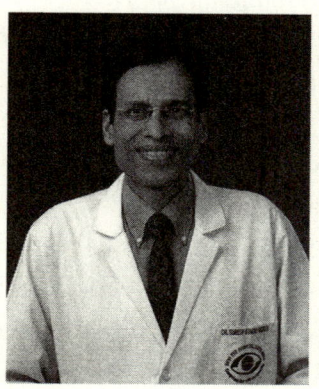

Dr Suresh K. Pandey is an author, world-renowned eye surgeon, and Director of the SuVi Eye Hospital & Lasik Laser Centre, Kota, Rajasthan, India. He is a member of the prestigious International Intraocular Implant Club (IIIC). He is the former vice president of the Indian Medical Association (IMA) Kota and the former president of the Kota Division Ophthalmological Society (KDOS), Kota. Dr Pandey completed his ophthalmology residency from the prestigious Post Graduate Institute of Medical Education & Research (PGIMER), Chandigarh, and pursued an anterior segment fellowship in the USA and Australia. He has also performed live surgeries at various national and international conferences and has received several awards including Achievement Award (American Academy of Ophthalmology), Best-of-Show Video Award, Best Poster Award, Best-Paper-of-the-Session Award, etc. at the American Academy of Ophthalmology (AAO), American Society of Cataract and Refractive Surgery (ASCRS), Asia Pacific Association of Cataract and Refractive Surgeons (APACRS), European Society of Cataract and Refractive Surgeons (ESCRS) International Conferences and was awarded a Gold Medal by the Indian Intraocular Implant and Refractive Surgery Society. His three books, *Secrets of Successful Doctors: A Complete Guide Fulfilling Medical Career*, and *A Hippocratic Odyssey: Lessons from a Doctor Couple on Life in Medicine, Challenges, and Doctorpreneurship, Entrepreneurship for Doctors* continue to be popular among medical professionals. Dr Pandey's hobbies include cycling, painting, gardening, and photography.

Dr Suresh K. Pandey can be reached at:
E-mail: suresh.pandey@gmail.com
Phone Number: +919351412449
Twitter: https://twitter.com/SuViEyeKOTARAJ
Facebook: https://www.facebook.com/drsureshpandey
Instagram: https://www.instagram.com/drsureshkpandey/
LinkedIn: https://www.linkedin.com/in/eyedrsureshkpandeykota/
Website: www.drsureshpandey.com, www.suvieyehospital.com

Scan QR code to access the
Penguin Random House India website